# Green Candles

The easy way to make
Healthy &
Environmentally Friendly
Candles

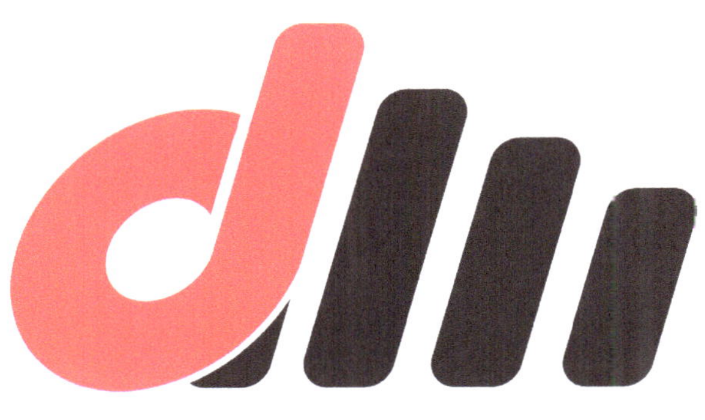

Dennis&Matt

# Green Candles

## The easy way to make Healthy & Environmentally Friendly Candles

---

Published by Lulu.com



Cover illustration by adsolutions

ISBN: 9781676619533

A Publication by

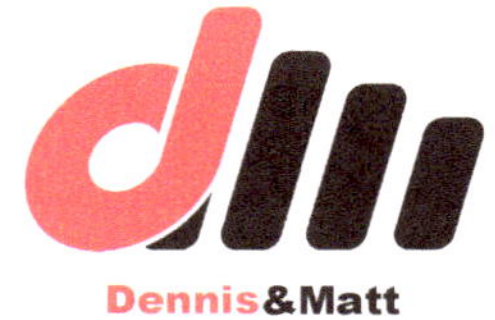


Bibra Lake, Western Australia 6163

www.yy157570.com

# Table of Contents

# History

Candle making was developed in many countries throughout history. The Egyptians formed candles that were made out of beeswax as early as 3000 BC. The Chinese created candles from whale fat during the Qin Dynasty 221 – 206 BC. In early China and Japan, tapers were made with wax from insects and seeds, wrapped in paper. In India, wax from boiling cinnamon was used for temple candles. During the first century AD, indigenous people of the Pacific Northwest fused oil from the eulachon, or candlefish, forlighting.

### 1500 AD to the present

During the middle ages in Europe, the popularity of candles is shown by their use in Candlemas and St Lucy festivities. Tallow, fat from sheep and cattle, became the standard material used in candles in Europe. The Tallow Candle Company of London was formed in about 1300, and in 1484 was granted a coat of arms. By 1415, tallow candles were used as street lighting. The unpleasant smell of tallow candles was due to the glycerin they contained. Churches and royal events used candles made out ofbeeswax as the smell was usually less unpleasant.

In 1750 oil from the sperm whale was used to provide very expensive candles. By 1800, a much cheaper wax derived from plant material was discovered, which yielded candles that produced clear and smokeless flames. Stearin was patented in 1611 by two French chemists. Like tallow, this was derived from animals, but had no glycerin in it.

Despite advances in candle making, the candle making industry was devastated by the distillation of kerosene (also known as paraffin oil or paraffin); this had little to do with paraffin wax. From here on the candles became more of a decorative item rather than a necessity.

It was during the 19th century when most of the major developments affecting candle making occurred. In 1834 inventor Joseph Morgan introduced a machine which did continuous production of molded candles. This machine extruded the candle as itcooled and solidified.

Increasing developments in candle making with the production of paraffin wax from oil and coal shale and processed by distilling the residues left from refining crude petroleum, the bluish white wax was found to burn cleanly and had no unpleasant smell. Of most importance was that the low cost compared to all preceding candle production. Although paraffin wax's low melting point may have imposed a threat to its popular use, the discovery of a compound (stearic acid) for hardening it solved the problem. By the end of the 19th century most candles consisted of paraffin wax and stearic acid.

No longer a major source of light, candles continue to grow in popularity and use. Today, candles are used for celebration, romance, ceremonies and accent décor.

There are more than 300 known commercial, religious and institutional manufacturers of candles in the US alone, as well as many small craft producers for local use.

Prior to the advent of clocks and watches candles were used to tell the time. People found that candles would burn at a set rate depending on the type and diameter of the candle, making them perfect for calculating the passing hours.

More recently, instead of lighting, candles have been used for meditation, aromatherapy, and other refreshing scents, to exude perfume through the home or workplace.

# Types and Uses of Candle Wax

There are many different types of candle wax. There are cheap candle waxes and there are costly waxes that are made into candles with slower melting rates.

There are different waxes blended in some candles, and some of these waxes have other uses. Listed below are some of the different types of waxes that are commonly used in candle making:

- Paraffin Wax:

  - A wax made of paraffin is a chemical preservative that is used commonly on fruit, vegetables, and sweets. This is in order to create a shiny appearance, delay the moisture loss and reduce spoilage. Chocolate makers quite often use paraffin wax. Paraffin wax is also known as "canning or baker's wax".

  - Paraffin wax is very flammable therefore make sure that you do not overheat it. Use a double boiler or microwave and heat it to the point of where the wax has dissolved (48 -65 deg C)

**The Dangers of Burning Paraffin Candles:**
If you burn paraffin candles, you might as well be inhaling diesel fumes. "The fine particulate matter collected from candle emissions was similar to that of diesel engine exhaust in particle size, morphology, elemental carbon content, and absorbed chemical constituents" says David Krause. Krause is an air quality engineer and former employee of the Florida Department of Health. He also adds, "These similarities point to a similar potential for adverse health effects."

These chemicals are also normally found in paraffin candles:

Acrolein, formaldehyde and acetaldehyde exceeding EPA safety thresholds, dibutyl phthalate, diethyl phthalate, bis (2-ethylhexyl) phthalate, didecyl phthalate, toluene, styrene, benzene, styrene, toluene, ethyl benzene, naphthalene, benzaldehyde, benzene;ethanol, and 2-butanone (methyl ethyl ketone) and acetone.

With the craze for gel candles you can add in mineral oil, terpene-type chemicals, modified hydrocarbons & viscosity increasing chemicals.

- Soy Wax:

  - Soy wax was discovered around the late 19th century and it was in the 1990s that "Michael Richards" searched to find a cheaper product than beeswax. It was he that developed and put soy wax on the market. In late 1996, he succeeded in changing from the costly beeswax to soy and palm wax. This wax is mainly used for container candles.

- Beeswax:

  - Beeswax is a natural wax, created by young worker bees.

  - Palm wax: Palm wax is made from natural palm oil. This wax has been around for a very long time. It has been grown, cultivated and harvested in Asia for at least 200 years. The palm wax is unlike other waxes as they form crystal-like substances on the outer side of the candle. Palm wax burns at a lot cooler and slower rate than a lot of other waxes

  - Palm wax is biodegradable and water soluble. The candles burn approximately 45 percent longer compared to paraffin candles of comparable size. Palm wax candles take up more scent than any other candle wax and the scent does not fade away like other candles.

  - This wax is great for pillar candles as it is a very sturdy wax. It blends well with other waxes, takes on dyes and scents very well and has an excellent throw. (i.e. distance that the scent can be smelt from the candle)

  - This wax has many uses and is used in the manufacturing of cosmetics, lotions, soaps balms and other products.

## Candle Wax, and Your Health

Candle wax has gone through lots of changes over time. From being made out of crude oil products, insects, animal fats, plants and other oils.

We need to focus on the healthy waxes rather than on any of the petroleum type waxes.

You have to be very careful when purchasing an all-natural wax candle. If it doesn't state all natural wax, 100% soy wax, natural wax blend, soy vegetable wax blend, 100% palm wax 100% beeswax or 100% bayberry wax then you are more likely not getting an all-natural wax.

Remember the wax is a vapor that actually burns along with the scent oil. So, if you are using petroleum based waxes then you will get all the dangerous fumes that they emit. Stick to the natural waxes that way you will not have to worry.

## General Wax Instructions

**Heating, Processing, Mixing and pouring Wax:**

Place the candle wax in the pouring or wax heater and heat it until it is completely liquefied. Heating the candle wax up to 200 degrees F (93.33 °C) is generally fine. It is suggested that you add the colour and additives to your wax right around 190 degrees F (87.78 °C). Fully agitate it for several minutes, this will ensure that the wax has an even temperature throughout and the mix is blended thoroughly. Turn your heating unit down and let the wax cool to the recommended pouring temperature. We suggest adding the fragrance just before pouring: this avoids prolonged heating of the fragrance, which may contribute to some fragrance loss. It is imperative to agitate once again before pouring into the mould or containers. We can't stress enough the importance of pouring at correct temperature, pouring too hot may cause excessive shrinkage which may cause you to have to do multiple re-pours. On the other hand pouring too cool may cause unwanted air bubbles, blemishes and other defects on your candle's finish. Pouring at the incorrect temperature can also make it extremely difficult to get the candle out of the mould.

Once you have the initial pour done, your work is not over. It is a typical property of wax to shrink when cooled, which may require you to do a re-pour. There are certain container candle wax blends that may not need a re-pour. Typically, most waxes do require a re-pour or top-up. Make sure you save enough wax from the original batch so the colour of the top-up is consistent with the first pour. With container waxes we suggest letting the wax completely solidify before the re-pour. This will help you keep it to one top-up. In pillar and votive candles it may require some experimenting but we suggest waiting only an hour or two before re-pouring. Many times if you wait too long the wax will begin to shrink and pull away from the top of the mould. This will be a problem on the top—up, because when you do the top-up the molten wax will run down the side causing unwanted wax streaks on your candle's finish.

**Mould or Container Preparations:**

Whether you are making container candles, votives and/or pillar candles we suggest that you pre- heat your moulds of containers. A cold mould or container may cause surface chilling on your candle. Heating them will help you obtain a very smooth and clean finish on your candle. It is also suggested that you use some type of silicone mould release every 4 – 5 pours in your mould; this will ensure that you will have no difficulties in getting your candle out.

**Cooling:**

Depending on your wax formula or type of finish you are trying to achieve on your finished candle, you will need to consider the cooling method. Candles may be cooled at room temperature or forced cooled by circulating air, refrigeration, or cold water baths. If you are making container candles, we suggest letting the candle cool at ambient temperature to help minimise shrinkage. Force cooling candles usually results in separation between the wax and the glass causing undesirable wet spots.

# Candle Wicks

No wicks no candles!!

Candle wicks have fibres mostly cotton; these fibres are braided into several different thicknesses. Basically three different styles or types are used with different candles. The three styles are: Flat, Square and Cored.

### Cored wicks

The wicks can be all cotton or they can be cored, meaning they have something in the middle of the wick. The wick can have anything from lead, zinc or paper in it. Back in the late 80's American manufacturers self-regulated and quit using lead cored wicks. However, lead cored wicks were still being imported into America from other countries. Australia was the first country to ban the importation of lead wicked candles. America and Canada soon followed with the ban. Sadly with the love for cheap products including candles the large discount and dollar stores still import almost all their candles and the only label is a little warning on the bottom and a name on the front.

Check the wick on the candle by poking with your fingernail and see if there is a wire in the wick, if there is then ask the store owner if it is lead. If he cannot answer then leave the candle alone. It may be zinc or tin, which are proven quite safe, but you will never know it may be LEAD.

The label has no information, where it was made, what is the wax. Place it back on the shelf, leave it alone. The company is trying to make a dollar off the uninformed customer and not caring about the customer's health.

### So what to do?

The best thing to do is to just buy candles from manufacturers that use all cotton candle wicks. All cotton as in ALL COTTON, or hemp cored wicks, which is a natural fibre with no unhealthy after affects. Or if they are zinc cored, ask the manufacturer, if the zinc is a good grade of zinc. The purer the better! Email or get information off the web. If they don't say just pass up. If they state that it's all cotton with a hemp core or even an all hemp wick, then it's OK.

### Wick size

A wick is sized for the size of the candle. If the wick is too large, the flame will be too large and overheat the candle wax. If the wick is too small it will tunnel down till it drowns, and you end up with a half burnt candle. If you dig the wick out of the wax and relight, it will only tunnel again.

Cotton Square Braid Wicks. Use for: most Pillar Candles, Dipped Candles (tapers)

| WICK SIZE | POOL DIAMETER | FLAME HEIGHT | BURNING SPEED *Grams per Hour* *(Ounces per Hour)* |
|---|---|---|---|
| 4/0 | 1.9" (48.26mm) | 1.3" (33.02mm) | 5.6g (0.20) |
| 3/0 | 2.0" (50.8mm) | 1.4" (35.56mm) | 6.2g (0.22) |

| | | | |
|---|---|---|---|
| 2/0 | 2.0" (50.8mm) | 1.5" (38.1mm) | 5.9g (0.21) |
| 1/0 | 2.2" (55.88mm) | 1.8" (45.72mm) | 7.0g (0.25) |
| #1 | 2.4" (60.96mm) | 1.7" (43.18mm) | 7.3g (0.26) |
| #2 | 2.4" (60.96mm) | 1.8" (45.72mm) | 7.3g (0.26) |
| #3 | 2.4" (60.96mm) | 1.9" (48.26mm) | 8.1g (0.29) |
| #4 | 2.4" (60.96mm) | 2.4" (60.96mm) | 8.7g (0.31) |
| #5 | 2.2" (55.88mm) | 2.8" (71.12mm) | 9.8g (0.35) |
| #6 | 2.2" (55.88mm) | 2.8" (71.12mm) | 10.1g (0.36) |
| #7 | 3.4" (86.36mm) | 3.2" (81.28mm) | 12.0g (0.43) |
| #8 | 2.2" (55.88mm) | 3.1" (78.74mm) | 10.9g (0.39) |
| #10 | 1.9" (482.6mm) | 3.5" (88.9mm) | 12.6g (0.45) |

**LX Coated Wick Assemblies** (wick tab attached). Use for: the wick of choice for Container candles, Tea-lights, Votives. Also suitable for Pillar candles.

| **WICK SIZE** | **POOL DIAMETER** | **FLAME HEIGHT** | **BURNING SPEED** ***Grams per Hour*** *(Ounces per Hour)* |
|---|---|---|---|
| LX10 | 2.0" (50.8mm) | 1.1" (27.94mm) | 4.2g (0.15) |
| LX12 | 2.1" (53.34mm) | 1.2" (30.48mm) | 5.0g (0.18) |
| LX14 | 2.1" (53.34mm) | 1.3" (33.02mm) | 5.3g (0.19) |
| LX16 | 2.2" (55.88mm) | 1.4" (35.56mm) | 5.6g (0.20) |

**Zinc Core Wicks**. Use for: Container Candles, Tea-Lights, Votives, Multi-Wicked Pillar Candles. Provides the most rigidity and coolest flame of all "Cored" wicks.

| **WICK SIZE** | **POOL DIAMETER** | **FLAME HEIGHT** | **BURNING SPEED** ***Grams per Hour*** *(Ounces per Hour)* |
|---|---|---|---|
| 44-24-18 Z | 2.0" (50.8mm) | 1.0" (25.4mm) | 4.2g (0.15) |
| 60-44-18 Z | 2.3" (58.42mm) | 1.7" (43.18mm) | 6.4g (0.23) |

When your candles burn down to the tabs and leave that 6mm of wax on the bottom, use a knife to chunk it up and then use them in a melter, this allows you to get the rest of the perfume out of the wax.

If the wicks get too long, cut them back to around 6mm. The perfect candle needs very little trimming. It is best to use a candle wick trimmer as they have a little plate to catch the trimming.

If you use scissors remove the trimming from the candle before lighting, otherwise you will get improper burning.

To get the most out of your candle if it's a container candle, burn it till you have a complete pool of wax on the top. Then let it rest and light another one. This way your candle will last longer.

### Always use a snuffer

The snuffer helps keep your wick from smoking after you put it out.

If you blow it out, even if it's an all-cotton or hemp wick and the best candle on the market, the wick will smoke. By using the snuffer you push the wick into the liquid wax and drown it, and also put wax on the wick tip thus allowing easier lighting next time. Just ensure that you straighten the wick once it goes out. Use the snuffer to lift it out of the wax.

By using the proper selection and care of your wicks you will get the most out of every candle. Always ensure that you put the candles in a place where there are no drafts. Don't place the candles close any drapes or clothing as they may contact the flame. Always put the candles on a plate or tray to ensure that if any spill occurs the wax will not cause either damage to the article it is on or create a flare up.

## Scented oils for candle

In history we learnt how the first fragrance oils came into being. They were made from seeds, bathing oils, nuts, insects and fruits. The essential oils were made from herbs, plants, flowers and other natural products. These were also added to candle wax to scent them. These were the first aromatherapy candles.

### Fragrance oils or Essential oils

These two oils were followed by third oil which is synthetic fragrances. Synthetic oils are a large part of the fragrance industry. Synthetic oils give some of the most unique fragrances for scented oil candles. However, you need to stay clear of anything synthetic in Essential Oils; these oils need to be pure to be fully effective.

An **essential oil** is a concentrated, hydrophobic liquid containing volatile aroma compounds from plants. They are also known as **volatile** or **ethereal** oils, or simply as the "oil of" the plant material from which they were extracted, such as *oil of clove.* Oil is "essential" in the sense that it carries a distinctive scent, or essence, of the plant. Essential oils do not as a group; need to have any specific chemical properties in common, beyond conveying characteristic fragrances. They are not to be confused with essential fatty acids.

Essential oils are generally extracted by distillation. Other processes include expression, or solvent extraction. They are used in perfumes, cosmetics and bath products, for flavoring food and drink, and for scenting incense and household cleaning products.

Various essential oils have been used medicinally at different periods in history. Medical applications proposed by those who sell medicinal oils range from skin treatments to remedies for cancer, and are often based on historical use of these oils for these purposes. Such claims are now subject to regulation in most countries, and have grown correspondingly more vague, to stay within these regulations.

Interest in essential oils has revived in recent decades, with the popularity of aromatherapy, a branch of alternative medicine which claims that the specific aromas carried by essential oils have curative effects. Oils are volatilized or diluted in carrier oil and used in massage, or burned as incense.

Fragrance oil (s), also known as **aroma oils**, **aromatic oils**, and **flavour oils**, are blended synthetic aroma compounds or natural essential oils that are diluted with a carrier like propylene glycol, vegetable oil, or mineral oil. Aromatic oils are used in perfumery, cosmetics, flavoring of food, and in aromatherapy

Synthetic fragrance oils are used because they are more affordable than pure unadulterated essential oils. The majority of adverse reactions to cosmetics and toiletries are caused by fragrance chemicals. Most hypo-allergenic forms of cosmetics are fragrance free because the chemical cocktails are known irritants and allergens. The consumer has such negative reactions to cosmetic fragrances because each artificial fragrance typically contains one hundred or more chemicals to produce just one fragrance. Over 5000 aroma chemical are available for creating synthetic fragrances.

On the other hand, essential oils are highly concentrated and potent oils extracted from plants, leaves, flowers, roots, buds, twigs, rhizomes, heartwood, bark, resin, seeds and citrus fruits. According to the International Organization for Standardization, essential oils are a natural "product made by distillation with either water or steam or by mechanical processing of citrus rinds or by dry distillation of natural materials. Following the distillation, the essential oil is physically separated from the water phase." The water phase, which is the by product is then sold as hydrosols or distillate waters. Each essential oil comes from just one source, a living plant. There are no chemicals involved. For the safest essential oils it is best to buy organic or wild craft essential oils so that no chemicals or pesticides ever entered the life cycle of the plant source of the essential oil.

It is unhealthy to buy products that contain anything other than pure unadulterated essential oils or distillate waters, no matter how attracted to the synthetic fragrance that you may be. By law you can claim that you use "essential oils" even if you use "reconstitutes, nature identicals, isolates, perfume compounds, aromas, synthetic fragrance or diluted essential oils." It is legal to claim that you only use essential oils, when in fact you add synthetics in your product, but it is unscrupulous. Read you labels carefully an d make sure that only Essential Oils, Distillate Waters or Hydrosols are listed in the ingredient list and never "Fragrance", "Fragrance Oils", "Perfume" or "Parfum". The best way to know the difference, so that even a poorly labeled product will not sneak past you, is to educate you nose by smelling essential oils next to fragrance oils. Once you smell the difference you will never be misled again. Nothing man made smells as perfect and just like the fresh cut plant as a true essential oil or distillate water.

# Types and Using Dyes in candles

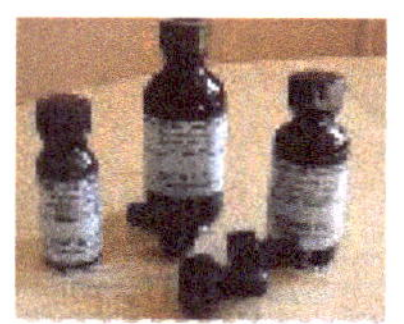

### Candle Making Liquid Dye

Candle making liquid dyes (oil based) are more potent than other types of dye, and a little dye (a couple of drops) goes a long way. Liquid dyes work really well with gel candles, and you can make darker or richer colors by mixing in a little black dye. Liquid dyes also mix better in soy wax than other types of dyes. This dye is made specifically for Candle Making and will not clog wicks when burning.

1 ounce of dye will color approximately 62 pounds of wax. Some darker colors color less than 62 pounds depending on your formula and scent. Dyes are packaged by weight not volume,

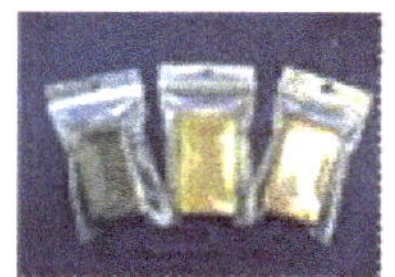

### Candle Making Dye Blocks

Candle Coloring - These 1/2 oz. dye blocks are highly concentrated candle dyes. One dye block will color 15 to 20 of pounds of Paraffin, Gel or Soy wax. You should only use a small sliver at a time (potato peelers are great!) until the desired color is achieved as you can always add more dye - but you can't take it out!

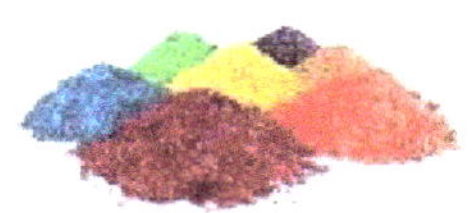

### Fluorescent Pigment dye flakes

This range of dyes are classified as pigments so cannot be used like normal dye blocks or liquid dyes. Pigments are great for over dipping or adding with your existing dyes for a brighter, sharper glow to your existing colours.

Pigments can clog the wicks so usage is recommended at **no more than 0.5% and extensive testing is a must.**

# Primary Colors - how they Work

When you work with color, two of the most important things to learn are:

1. How to mix colors so that you can get exactly what you want.
2. How to control color values so that your pictures don't look too flat.

Primary means "first," and primary colors are therefore the first colors you need in order to mix a variety of other colors. Knowing your primary colors is the first step to achieving proper color mixing.

### What are primary colors?

Color is actually a component of light. Light travels in waves, and these waves have different lengths and speeds. When the waves reach our visual receptors (our eyes), we experience the sensation of color. These wavelengths of light can be broken down into three (primary) categories:

1. The longer, slower wavelengths produce red light.
2. The shorter, quicker wavelengths produce blue light.

3. The middle range wavelengths produce green light.

An equal mixture of these wavelengths produces pure white light.

Red, green and blue are called the primary colors of light. These colors are used to project images in television screens, computer monitors, and anything that transmits light from a light source.

But, as artists, we are using pigments (paints, inks, dyes, etc.), not light. So what does light have to do with primary colors? Actually, everything! Colors of pigment are produced by reflecting and absorbing certain wavelengths of light.

**Primary Colors of Pigment**

A primary color of pigment is a color that reflects equal parts of any two of the (primary) colors of light (red, green and blue). (Diagram A, which can be viewed online at www.colorwheelco.com/use_cmywheel.html, illustrates the result of projecting red, green and blue lights onto a white surface in overlapping fashion.) Where any one light reaches the surface, it is reflected back from the surface. Where two lights overlap, they are both reflected from the surface, resulting in a mixture of those two colors. Here's how it works:

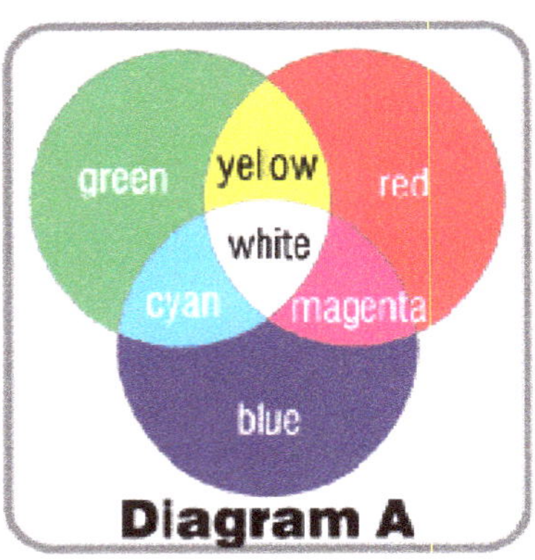

Diagram A

- Where red and blue lights overlap, they combine to produce magenta.
- Where blue and green lights overlap, they combine to produce cyan.
- Where green and red lights overlap, they combine to produce yellow.

And where all three lights overlap, they combine to produce white.

These three resulting colors--cyan, magenta and yellow--are the three primary colors of pigment. These are the purest colors and cannot be produced by mixing other pigment colors. Using these three colors, you can produce a vast number of other colors. When white or black are added to your colors, the range is even greater.

Following is a very basic guide for mixing colors using cyan, magenta and yellow:

**Mixing Colors**

First, let's take a look at what happens when we overlap the three primary colors of pigment. Using a format similar to Diagram A, we can mix "equal" parts of any two of these primary colors to produce an opposite result. Diagram B at illustrates the results of blending (mixing) equal parts of any two primary colors of pigment. Because pigments reflect and absorb light, their resulting mixtures are not as pure as light.

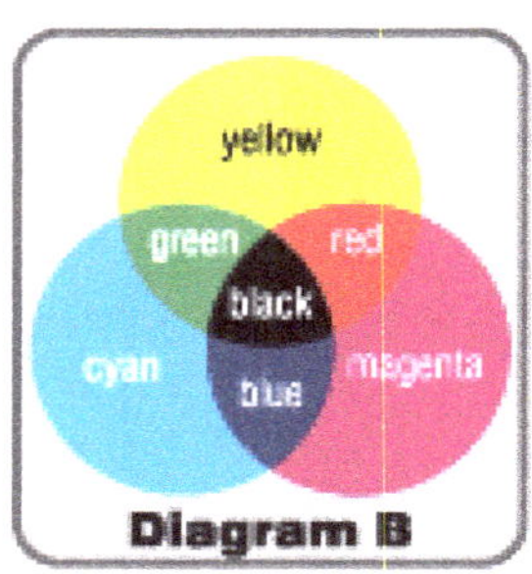

Diagram B

Some pigments tend to be more intense than others, so an "equal" mixture is relative to the intensity of the pigment. This is why a color wheel is very useful as a guide to color matching.

When magenta and cyan pigments are blended, the resulting mixture is blue. When cyan and yellow pigments are blended, the resulting mixture is green. When yellow and magenta pigments are blended, the resulting mixture is red. When all three colors are blended, the result is a "black" color.

This black is rarely a pure black, as some light is still being reflected. Okay, so now we have our three primary colors. How can we produce so many other colors from just these three? Actually color is quite mathematical. Just as you can add 1 and 1 to make 2, or 0.5 and 0.5 to make 1, you can mix colors in a similar manner. Let's start with yellow and magenta. If you mix these two colors together, you produce red. What would happen if you then mix yellow and red? Here you have twice as much yellow as magenta, and the resulting color is orange. Diagram C, shows how colors can be incrementally mixed to produce a vast array of "in-between colors.

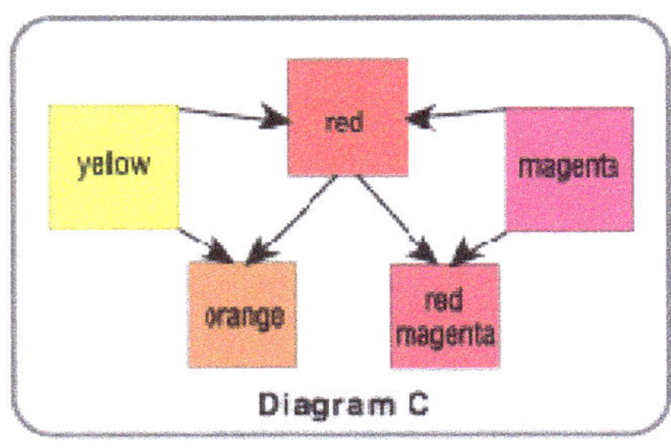

Diagram C

But what if you want to produce a beautiful, rich brown, a maroon, or a subtle grayish-blue? This is where placing colors around a wheel is an excellent way to illustrate color mixtures. The colors we have looked at so far are produced in a "linear" fashion, by mixing any two colors equally, then varying the amount of each of the two primary colors. If we look at colors arranged in a circle, we will see that colors can also be mixed across the circle. So far, we have mixed only around the outside of the circle.

**Creating Tones**
"Breaking colors" across the wheel, or creating tones, is achieved by mixing varying amounts of colors that are opposite each other on the color wheel. For instance, if you mix equal parts of red and cyan (opposite colors or complements), the result will be a dark grayish-black color. (Opposite colors neutralize each other.) If you mix a small part of cyan to red, the result will be a red-brown color. If you mix more cyan, the result will be a bit grayer, etc. When creating tones, you are actually lowering the saturation, or intensity, of the original pure colors.

**Creating Tints**
When you add white to a color, you are creating a tint of that color. The more white you add, the lighter the color becomes.

**Creating Shades**
When you add black to a color, you are creating a shade of that color. The more black you add, the deeper the color becomes.

**Start Mixing**

Now you have the basics of mixing colors from the three primary colors--cyan, magenta and yellow. If you have a color wheel, it will be easier to practice mixing, as you can look at the wheel and have an actual color to match. Practice mixing colors around the wheel, and when you are happy with the results, try mixing across the wheel, then creating tints and shades by adding white or black to any of your colors. Happy painting!

# Containers

What constitutes a container? Well, just about any container the right size for the candle you are making will do. As long as it does not melt, burn, leak or crack with the heat.

Moulds can be made out of metal, plastic, rubber, silicone, cardboard or clay. Some of these will need to be sealed prior to pouring of the wax. They can be of any shape or size. Again so long as you can remove the candle from them without damaging the candle once it has cooled. For the more intricate type moulds you will need to have a two piece metal or plastic mould or rubber / silicone type mould which can be split and spread to remove from the candle.

Here are a few designs and types of moulds that are available on the market:

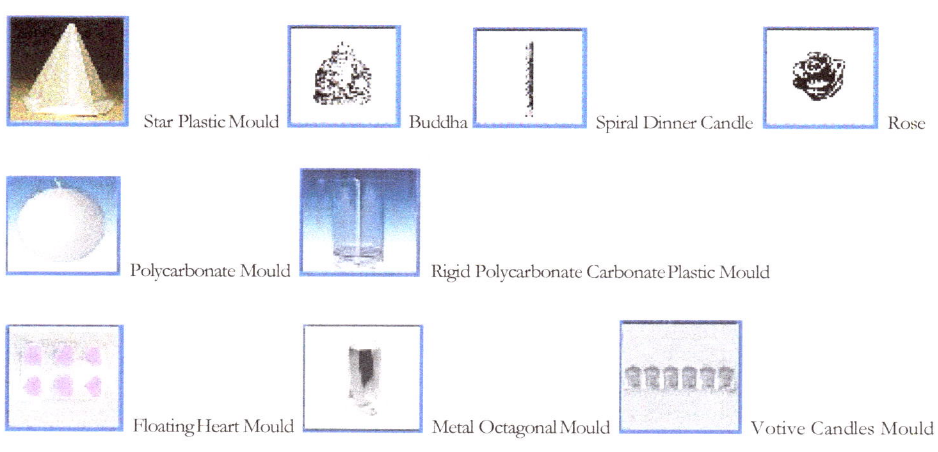

Star Plastic Mould Buddha Spiral Dinner Candle Rose

Polycarbonate Mould Rigid Polycarbonate Carbonate Plastic Mould

Floating Heart Mould Metal Octagonal Mould Votive Candles Mould

**Votive Candle Holders**

Make sure that the votive candle holders are made to burn votives. (Not shot glasses or any other little glasses as they may notwithstand the heat).

Make sure that the votive fits tightly and isn't larger than the container. If you are making your candles then the good thing about votive candle holders is that you can stick pre-tabbed wicks in the bottom and pour any leftover from your pouring to use as samples or to give away as a gift.

You can also use any of your jar candles that are at the finish of their life and would have been tossed. Whilst they are still molten just pour it into the prepared votive holder and you have a nice little scented candle.

Or, if the container candle goes out and there is still some left in the bottom them just chip it out and use the chips in a candle warmer

**What constitutes a Safe Container?**

Use only safe containers for pouring container candles. There are at least two categories of containers that could be considered unsafe. They are ones that are prone to cracking and the other is the one that has the potential to act as a wick.

Porous materials such as clay flower pots, any unsealed earthen ware can act as a wick. It is possible for the clay pot to wick the molten wax through the pot and draw enough wax to fuel the combustion cycle of the flame. Therefore the normal flame of about 25mm could be increased to the entire width of the pot. This is a rare occurrence. However, it is possible.

The container that is prone to cracking can pose a risk either when pouring the wax or when burning. Where the container cracks whilst pouring will spill all over the place. Therefore you need to wear shoes and other protective clothing when pouring. The more dangerous condition exists when the container cracks whilst burning and allows the wax to spill all over the place. This in turn exposes an increase of wick and therefore rapid increase in flame length, which in turn could catch hold of any flammable material near it.

A number of things can be done to prevent cracked container candles. You can select glass and ceramic containers that are intended to withstand heat. You can select the smallest wick size that will produce the lowest amount of heat but sufficient for a decent melt pool. Make sure that the wick is properly centered to prevent the heat buildup with localised area of the glass. Or, use low melting point waxes to help keep them cool.

Flame surge from freshly exposed wick can occur with any kind of candle. A votive that has fully liquefied could crack the glass and suddenly expose the wick, or a pillar that has been burning for a long period of time could have one of its side crumble and expose the extra length of wick.

No matter what container made out of glass or ceramic is prone to cracking, even those stated as heat resistant, such as glassware made especially for candle making and canning jars. "I have even had a container with Pyrex written on it shatter on me when I applied heat to it (It was made in China)". The most important thing coming out of this is that all candles should be burnt on a heat resistant surface, under supervision and well away from any flammable material.

The likelihood of glassware or ceramic designed for heat cracking is minimal, however, users seeing these as proper candle holders could possible trust them fully. These then are the unsafe containers. Thus the only containers that are safe are the ones that are under full supervision.

# Safety

- ✓ Always keep a burning candle within sight. Extinguish all candles when you leave a room or go to sleep
- ✓ Never burn a candle near or on anything that can catch fire. Keep candles away from drapes, bedding, books, clothing, carpets and other flammable material and decorations.
- ✓ Keep out ofreach of children and pets.
- ✓ Do not place burning candles where they can be knocked over by anyone.
- ✓ Trim wicks to 6mm each time of lighting. Long or crooked wicks create uneven burning.
- ✓ Always use a proper candle holder designed for the candle. It should be large enough to contain the dripping of the candle wax and stable enough to not fall over easily.
- ✓ Ensure to read the instruction of the manufacturer fully and understand them
- ✓ Keep the burning candles away from drafts and vents as this will prevent uneven and rapid burning.
- ✓ Keep wax pool free of wick and match debris at all times.
- ✓ Do not burn candles longer than manufacturers recommendations
- ✓ Always burn candles in well ventilated room.
- ✓ Never touch or move a votive or container candle whilst it is still liquid.
- ✓ Extinguish pillar wax candles if the wax pool comes too close to the edge of the candle.
- ✓ Candles should be places at least 75mm apart from each other to ensure that they don't melt with the extra heat.
- ✓ One of the safest ways to extinguish a candle is with a candle snuffer.
- ✓ Do not extinguish candles with water as it can spatter and cause serious burns on contact. This also may cause the container to crack due to the difference in temperatures involved.
- ✓ Never use candles for light when refueling equipment such as a lantern or heater.
- ✓ Never use a lighted candle in confined spaces as it will burn up all the oxygen in the area.

- ✓ When breaking in your candle allow it to burn long enough on your first lightning to pool the wax to almost reaching the container. In future the candle will only burn to this area as they did the first time. Once broken in burn no longer than 2 hours at a time.

- ✓ Burn approximately one hour for each inch in diameter. The outer wall of the candle keeps the melted wax pool inside, but if a candle is left burning too long, the heat will extend to the outer wall and crack or melt it. (Paraffin wax would normally tend to melt, whereas palm wax is stronger, so it usually tends to crack instead). To extend the life of the candle, you would want to burn a 3" wide candle for approximately 3 hours, a 4" wide candle for 4 hours, etc. This is an average. Different conditions will always factor in, so it is best to always keep a close eye on the candle. In doing this, you will be able to judge when the wax pool is large enough that the candle should be blown out and allowed to cool down. A thin outer wall of the candle should be left behind as the candle burns down. This is normal, and not only helps keep the wax pool inside, but it also helps to create the soft flicking that most people desire when burning candles. I do not recommend trimming the candle wall unless it is cracked or becomes visually unappealing.

- ✓ Extinguish and dispose of pillar candles when they have less than 2" left at the bottom. When candles reach less than 2", they should no longer be used as candles. You can throw them away, or more recycle them, as I like to do. I break my leftover candle into wax chips (discarding the wick remnant), and place the wax chips in a bowl or saucer, and use them to scent my closets. You can also place them in a small cloth or organza bag, and use them to scent dresser drawers. Or, if you have a wax melter, potpourri melter, etc., you can add the wax chips to them.

- ✓ Store candles on their sides in a dark and cool dry place.

Candles can evoke special memories, and enhance everyday life. They are a source of light and delight when used properly. By following the simple steps above, we can extend the life of our candles and ensure a safe and happy burning experience.

# Equipment for making candles

Before you start making your candles, you will need some basic equipment and tools. These are readily available from craft shops, mail order or through the internet. Check the supplier reviews page for candle making suppliers who I can recommend. If you do not wish to spend too much initially, you will probably find that you already have most of the basic tools, or at least adequate alternatives.

## Essential Supplies

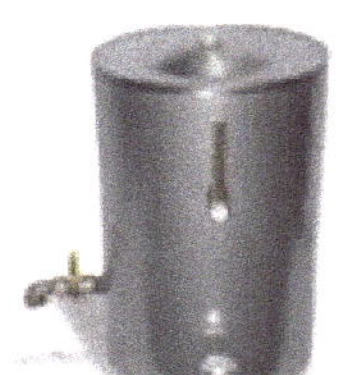

### Melting System

There are several methods of melting wax. DO NOT use a microwave or direct heat!! For a beginner I would recommend a double boiler system which is essentially two saucepans one inside the other. Fill the bottom pan 1/3 full of water and place the wax in the top one. Never leave a double boiler unattended as the water will quickly evaporate unless you keep topping it up as it needs. If the water runs out it can cause a fire hazard. Available worldwide is the Burco system which is essentially a big version of a double boiler except it has the temperature control. As you learn more about candle making you will learn why temperature is so important. See making your first candle to find out more about temperature. If you don't want to spend out on big melters, you can make do just as well with a coffee can set inside a saucepan 1/3 full of water.

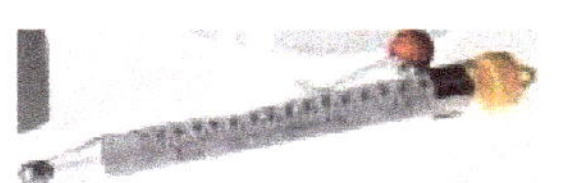

### Thermometer

To measure the temperature of your melting wax, a specialist thermometer covering the scale 38-177C (100-350F) is recommended. A candy thermometer covers the same scale. You cannot use a normal household thermometer as it does not go high enough. This is really an essential piece of equipment although your candles will burn fine without the use of a thermometer; it can solve a lot of troubleshooting problems with surface marks on your candles if you check the temperature of your wax before pouring into a mold.

### Scales

Required to measure the amount of wax and other materials you are using. Kitchen scales are ideal.

### Ladle

Handy to ladle the wax out of your melter.

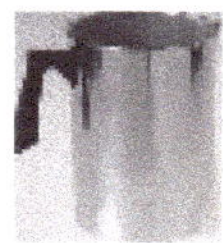

### Measuring /Pouring Jug

Ladle out your wax into a jug and use the jug to pour into the molds. It will be easier to control pouring into molds if you pour from a jug.

### Wax

A very essential part of candle making! You can't make candles without wax!! You've all heard the saying "you get what you pay for" so use a quality supplier rather than canning wax from the grocery store. Your candles will thankyou.

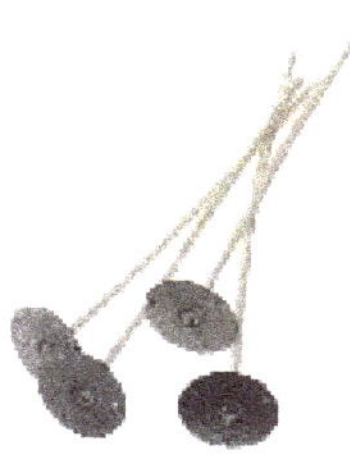

### Wick

Comes in all types and sizes depending on the project you are using. The most common suitable candle making wick is braided cotton that has been treated chemically to improve the quality of burning. Wick is sold in graduations and the size of your candle determines the size of the wick. If you are unsure, tell the supplier what size diameter candle you intend to make and they can recommend the correct wick for you.

**Colouring / Dye**

Used by candle makers to make a vast range of colours and shades. How much you use depends on the size of your candle and how dark. you want it to be. The more dye you use, the deeper the colour. Do not use wax crayons as it clogs the wick. Proper candle dyes are inexpensive and worth investing in. There are several different sorts of dyes blocks that you shave a small amount off of into the wax, colour chips which are smaller and work on the same principle as blocks or there are liquid dyes which are controlled by a dropper. To start with I would recommend blocks or chips in the basic primary colours, red, blue and yellow. You can make all the colours you need from these three and you can always invest in extra once you've got the hang of basic colour mixing. Candle dyes are available from all good suppliers.

**Wax Additives**

There are lots of different additives you can add to your wax to create different effects. The main two that you will need to start with are stearic acid (also known as stearin) and vybar. Stearin is a useful additive that increases the depth of the colours, reduces dripping and improves burning. It also increases the tendency of the paraffin wax to shrink, making removing candles from rigid moulds much easier. Use 10% of stearin to wax. Vybar increases the opacity (creaminess) of wax and helps it to burn better. Find out more about additives.

**Mold Seal**

If you plan on making pillar candles you will need something called mold seal to hold the wick in place so that the wax doesn't escape through the hole. Mould seal is similar to putty is re-useable and plumbers putty or blue-tack work great!

**Candle Molds**

Most candles are made from moulds, and these come in all shapes and sizes. Materials used include plastic, metal, rubber, latex and glass. The cheapest to start with are the basic plastic molds but you cannot use scent or high temperatures (wax over 180°F - 82 °C) in them. Metal molds are the most expensive but they are tough and sturdy and have the advantage of being suitable to heat before pouring the wax in to give a shiny finish to your candles. Novelty style candles with a lot of detail are generally made from 2 piece plastic or rubber. The shape of these enables you to make candles from odd shapes that could not be removed from a rigid straight mould. The main drawback to using a rubber or latex mould is that they have a limited lifespan. There are several household items that you can use to make your own molds when you are just starting out.

**Heat Gun / Blow Torch**

They can be used to cover up a multitude of sins as far as surface imperfections are concerned, use them to preheat metal molds before pouring wax in to keep the wax hot for as long as possible (makes the candle shiny) and also use them to get rid of bubbles in gel candles. In the Australia you can get a heat gun from Bunning's, Mitre Ten and similar places.

## Non Essential Supplies

### Wicking Needles

These are useful, but not essential to insert the wick into rubber/latex molds.

### Dipping Can

A tall cylindrical metal vessel used for making hand dipped tapers and over dipping molded candles. It must be deep and wide enough to allow a candle to be completely immersed. Professional dipping cans are made of metal and can be bought from craft shops or suppliers. A cheaper alternative if you are just starting out is a spaghetti boiler. These can be bought from kitchen shops. Again, they are non-essential for your first few candles.

### Water Bath

A water bath is essentially just a bucket of water. Put the freshly poured candle into a bucket and fill with water. Take care that water doesn't splash inside the mold and make sure the water level comes right up to the top of the mold. All these moulds and supplies are available commercially, either from your local craft shop, through mail order orby ordering online.

### Improvised Moulds & Equipment

- Jam / fruit tins, waxedmilk cartons,
- Poly pipe cut tolength,
- Wooden spoons, pegs, skewers, chopsticks and elasticbands,
- Homemade wick pins from coathangers,
- Masking tape, blue-tack,
- Aluminium foil, (used to cover burner and sealing the base of moulds) and
- Waxed paper sheet to place over your bench and other places that you don't want the wax to go on.

## Candle Making Vocabulary

**Back Fill / Topping Off –** With the exception of those blended waxes that have been designed as one-pour. All waxes have some level of shrinkage. As the candle sets up it will shrink around the middle of the candle requiring additional wax to be added. The back-fill / top-off will be necessary to create a smooth top in the containers or in the case of pillars a uniform bottom to the candle.

**Burn Rate** – The amount of wax that is consumed in 1 hour of burning with a specific wick. However, without some type of base the burn rate is difficult to evaluate

**Cored Wick** – This is any wick that has zinc, paper cotton or hemp in the middle to provide additional rigidity to the wick. Wicks such as flat braided, square braided and round wicks do not have any type of core.

**Scent Load** – This term especially relates to candle making. Generally it is the percentage of fragrance put in the wax. Scent load can be anywhere from 1percent – exceeding 10 percent in some instances. Ergo 28gr (1oz) of scent to 0.45kg (1lb) is equal to a 5 percent scentload.

**Fully refined Wax** – This is a wax that has been through the maximum refined process. A fully refined wax generally has a melt point of 52°C (125°F) or better and has lower oil content. The exact oil content will vary depending on the melt joint of the wax. Fully refined waxes are generally used to make pillars, votives and most candles other than containercandles.

**Needle Penetration** – This is commonly used to measure the hardness of the wax. While this is important when using waxes on high speed equipment and hand carved applications it is difficult to assess a wax on this merit alone.

**Melt Point** – This term is used to describe the diameter of liquid wax that occurs during the burning of the wick. In a 100mm (4") diameter glass the ideal situation is to get a melt pool as close as possible to the side of the container.

**Mottling** – This is a fracturing of the wax which will create a look on the exterior of the candle that is "whited out," snowflake looking or "washed out". This look has been made famous by several companies. Not all waxes are designed to mottle so be sure to choose a wax designed for that application.

**Mushrooming** – This is what can appear on top of the wick during the burning cycle. Basically, these are carbon deposits that build up on the wick. The following factors are some of the reasons why this can occur:

- The core of thewick
- Lack of oxygen (incontainers)
- Scent load and incorrect sizing of thewick.

Other factors can cause mushrooming, but these are the main causes. Mushrooming can cause excessive smoking and should be reduced as soon as possible.

**Natural wax** – At the present time there has been no clear cut definition assigned to this product as it relates to the candle industry. In general this is any wax that is a by-product of a plant, insect or other living creature.

**NST 2 Treatment** – Many of the natural waxes have a high acid level which can impact on the burning properties of many of the wicks. Wicks with this treatment allow them to perform in natural waxes.

**Polar / Non-polar** – These phrases generally apply when making gel candles and clear candles products. In order to be safe when using the references products a fragrance must be non-polar. In general non-polar fragrance means it will be compatible to the gel that it is going into. A polar fragrance can bleed out of the gel causing a safety concern when the candle is burned. If making paraffin candles this term is not really applicable.

**Polymers** – These products are used to increase the melt point of a wax, increase the vibrancy of the colours, improve opacity, or to 'strengthen' the wax. Common polymers include AC 400 and C
15. Many blended waxes will contain polymers.

**Pre-Wick Assembly** – Refers to a wick that is cut to a specific length, has a wax coating and a metal base.

**Scenti-Masterbatch** – Is a patented solid fragrance system. This system works best when using straight paraffin; and eliminates the need for other additives, and still gets large amounts of scent into the candle.

**Straight paraffin** – A standard wax that can be used in candles but does not contain any type of additives when sold. Many of the common waxes sold in craft stores and canning waxes are generally considered straight paraffins.

# How to Make the Candles

### Votive Candles

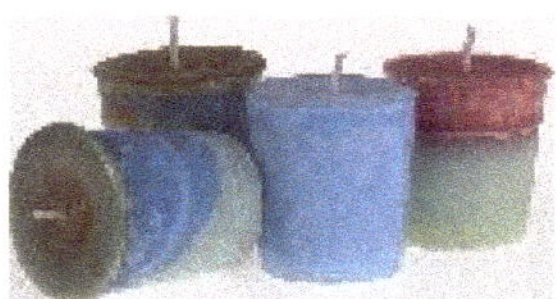

Votives are one of the easiest kinds of moulded candles to make. They add a great deal of charm to just about any setting. The typical votive candle will burn for approximately 15 hours and will consume just about all of the wax that was used to create it.

A properly crafted votive will liquefy to some degree as it burns. This is necessary to achieve good scent throw. Caution: Votives are not designed to be free standing. Therefore, it is important that votives are burnt in their proper holders.

What you will need:

- Wax suitable for votives
- Wax additives (only needed for your wax formulation)
- Fragrance oil (optional)

- Dye (Optional)
- Pre-tabbed wicks suitable for votives
- Votive moulds
- Mould release spray (optional)
- Pouring pot
- Thermometer

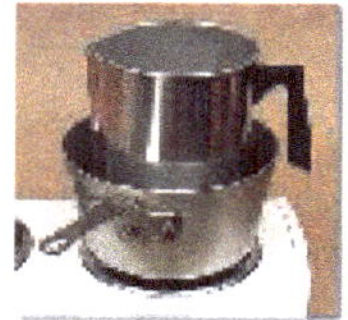

**Step 1. Prepare your melted wax mixture**. You should be able to review you're melting the wax. Before continuing, set up a double boiler to melt your wax. A good target temperature for votives is 80 °C (175 °F). Once your wax has completely melted add any additives you have selected and mix thoroughly, but try to avoid introducing air into the mixture, as it will possibly put little holes in the finished product.

Add the additives in the following order:

1. Additives such as vybar or stearic acid (stearin) (but only if needed)
2. Dye
3. Fragrance oil,(this is done last to avoid the loss of scent due to excess heating)

Before pouring the wax, you may want to lightly coat your moulds with a very thin film of mould release agent such as a silicone spray or cooking oil spray. This helps aid the release of the finished product from the mould. However, it is really only needed in new moulds.

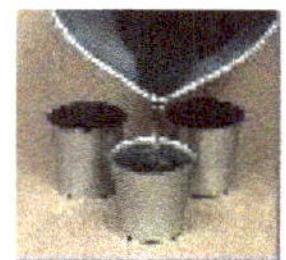

**Step 2. Votives: Initial Pour.** Place your votive moulds on a newspaper or greaseproof paper lined surface to catch any spills. With your wax at the proper pouring temperature about (80 °C (175 °F), fill your moulds to the lip of the mould. The objective here is to get the wax just up to the lip without overflowing. If you pour to a level lower than the lip, you may get seam lines in your finished candle.
Care should be taken to minimize the number of bubbles being introduced while pouring.

Save about 29 percent of your wax for the re-pour at a later step. Do not return it to the heat source, as it will lose some of the fragrance oil.

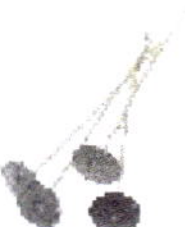

**Step 3. Add Pre-tabbed Wicks**. Wait for your wax to cool for a short time. While it is cooling, prepare your wicks by straightening them. They do not have to be perfectly straight at this time: a loose approximation of "straight" is fine.

Once the wax just begins to congeal, insert your pre-tabbed wicks. The tab will "stick" to the bottom when it touches. Care should be taken to position the tab roughly in the centre of the mould.

Why wait for the wax to begin congealing? You may well ask. At the temperature of the congealing point, the wax is cool enough that it will not interfere with the firmness of the primed wick. It also is the temperature that allows the metal tab the "stick" to the mould bottom. At higher temperatures, the wick can be a little more difficult to manage.

Once the tab has stuck to the base of the mould, it is very easy to straighten and manipulate the wick. Sometimes you may wish to wait a little longer to allow the metal tab to bond better before straightening the wick.

During the cooling process, the shrinking wax may pull the wick off centre. If this occurs, simply apply a light tug to straighten the wick. Do not use so much force as to free the metal tab from the bottom.

Allow the wax to cool down for an hour or so before going on to the next step.

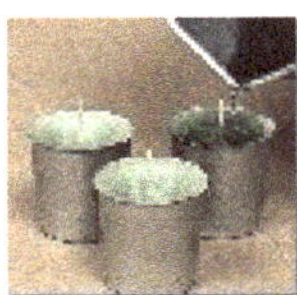

**Step 4. Re-pour Wax**. When the wax has cooled for an hour or two it will have shrunken a bit, leaving a sink hole that needs to be filled. Melt down the wax that you have saved from step 2 above. This time, your target pouring temperature will be 10 – 15 degrees hotter than the initial pour (88 °C – 190 °F). This increased temperature is to allow adhesion between the two layers.

Once the wax is at proper temperature, fill the moulds to a level slightly above the lip of the mould. Care should be taken to avoid spills.

Allow your candles to completely cool.

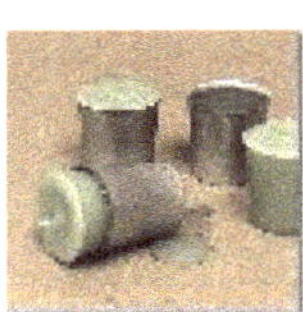

**Step 5. Remove Votive from Mould**. Once they are completely cool (3 -4 hours), remove them from the moulds. They usually slide right out without any difficulty if they are completely cool. If you attempt to take them out too soon, it will be more difficult to finally get them out.

If they are difficult to remove from the moulds, place them in the freezer for about 5 minutes and try again. If still difficult, then put them back for another 5 minutes.

Also, for very stubborn candles, it sometimes helps to gently press the sides of the mould inwards as you roll the mould in the palm of your hands.

## Making Pillar Candles

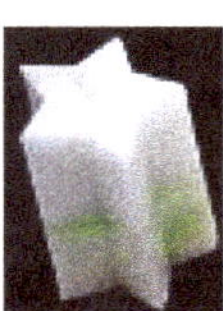

Moulded pillars are one of the most common types of candles we can make. There are many different shapes and sizes available to choose from. Aside from the different shapes and sizes, the moulds are fabricated out of sheet metal, aluminium, and even some are made of plastic, latex or silicone. The largest selection is typically available in sheet metal. Sheet metal and aluminium moulds are generally very durable and should last for years with very little maintenance.

The instructions presented here will use a mould fabricated from sheet metal. However, the procedure is the same for aluminium moulds. Please read the instructions for using plastic moulds as they will differ from plastic to plastic.

For wax selection, check the wax page. What you will need:

- Wax with any desired additives such as: dye, fragrance etc.
- Metal pillar mould
- Wick
- Wick screw
- Wick rod (or wooden skewer)
- Mould seal putty

**Step 1. Start by melting wax**. You should be able to review and carry out these instructions while your wax is melting. (Refer to double boiler instructions). Before continuing, set up a double boiler to melt your wax.

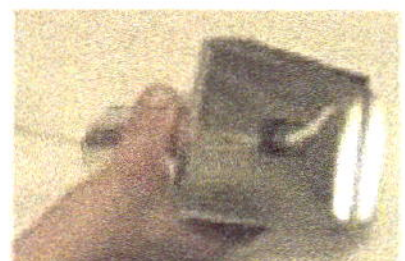

**Step 2. Press Wick through Wick Hole**. Select a wick of the proper size for the diameter of the mould you are working with (see table in wick page). Thread the wick through the wick hole in the base of the mould.

**Tip**: If it is difficult to get the wick through the hole because it is frayed then try dipping it in the molten wax and rolling it through your fingers to form a pointed end.

**Step 3. Secure Wick to Wick Rod.** While keeping the wick within the wick hole, tie one end of the wick to the wick rod. You can use a wooden skewer for this as the function is the same as a metal one.

**Step 4. Secure Wick to Wick Hole**. Secure the wick with a wick screw (usually provided by the manufacturer). Do not over tighten the wick screws it may cut the wick or damage the mould. The purpose of the wick screw is to simply keep the wick from sliding back through the hole, not to seal the hole (use mould sealer for that). Your wick should be taut, but do not tighten to the point where it will cause the mould to warp. Trim the wick leaving about 12mm – 25mm of wick. Use scissors or diagonal cutters for this.

Using some mould sealer, seal the wick hole, wick screw and wick. This is to stop leakage of the molten wax. Press the sealer firmly into place to ensure a tight seal. It may help to lightly wind the wick around the screw before applying the sealer. You don't want to be able to see any wick.

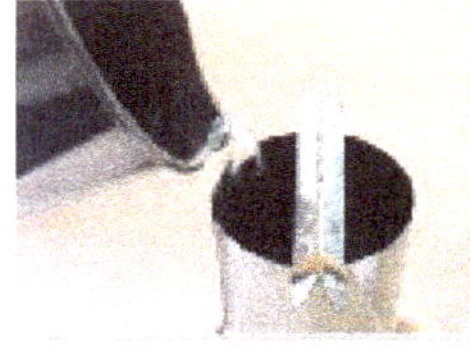

**Step 6. Initial Pour**. Once your wax has reached the proper temperature (175 - 185 °F / 80 °C – 85 °C for most pillars), add your additives (if any), your dyes and fragrance oil to the wax in the pouring pot and mix well using something such as a wooden spoon. Once it is thoroughly mixed, and is at the proper temperature, pour the wax into your prepared mould. Have an old towel or some paper towels to catch any spills that may occur. Fill your mould to about 12mm

from the top of the mould. Leave some wax in the pouring pot for later stage, but do not return it to the heat source yet.

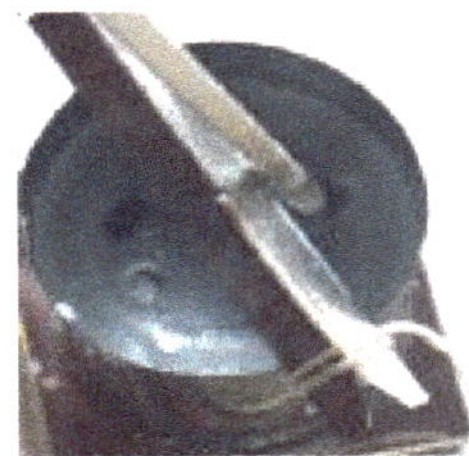

**Step 7. Poke Relief Holes**. Allow to cool a bit until a surface has formed on your wax. At this point poke relief holes into the base of the candle (at this point is the top of the candle) to accommodate the natural shrinkage that will occur as the wax solidifies. The relief holes should be positioned around the wick and should be poked to a depth of about 25mm less than the length of the candle. The exact number of holes is not important. The important thing is provide a vent by which the contacting volume of wax can suck air through to make up for the decreased volume. Without these relief holes, you may get air cavities within the candle, the wick may get pulled off centre, or the external walls of the candle may be deformed.

You may need to poke relief holes several times during the cooling process to ensure that the vent remains open and clear. Insuring that they are open will make it possible to fill in the voids on the next step.

Allow the candle to cool completely to room temperature before proceeding to the next step. This cooling process may take several hours. On very large candles, it may take in excess of a full day.

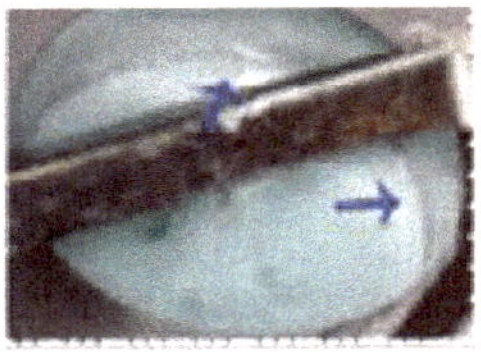

**Step 8. Re-pour to Fill in Void (sink hole).** Re-melt the leftover wax from step 6. This time you will need the temperature to be about 5 – 10 degrees hotter than the original pouring temperature. The hotter temperature aids adhesion between layers. Once, your wax is at the proper temperature, fill the sink holes in your candle. Fill to a level just below the level of the first filling. Filling higher than this may cause a horizontal seam line to be visible on the exterior of your finished candle. Over filling may also cause wax to seep down between the mould and the candle, resulting in an unsightly finish?

Allow the candle to cool completely before proceeding to the next step.

**Step 9. Remove Candle from Mould.** Remove the mould sealer and the wick screw. If cooled completely, your candle should slide out of the mould. If it does not slide out easily, then place candle in refrigerator for a period of about 15 minutes, then try again. The cooling will help the wax to shrink even more and help it separate from the mould.

The end of the candle attached to the wick rod is the bottom of the candle. Trim the wick flushes on this end.

If desired, you may level the base of the candle by placing the candle on a biscuit tray (one with sides works best) that is sitting on top of a pot of boiling water. Use the heated tray to melt away some of the wax until you have a flat base.

Trim the top wick to about 6mm. Your candle is now ready to be burned.

**Caution**: Burn pillars only on a designated candle holder.

## Making Floating Candles

Add beauty and elegance to any room with this easy project.

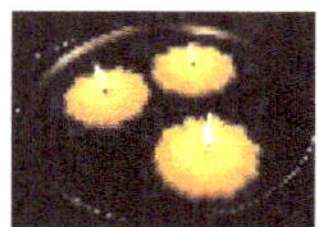

Any candle can actually be used as a floating candle, as long as it is wider than it is tall. Using proper floating moulds takes out all the guesswork and measurements required to help you create the perfect floating candle.

What you need:

- Any pillar wax or votive blend wax
- Floater mould
- Pre-tabbed wicks
- Pouring jug
- Your choice of fragrance oil and dye Creating floating candles is similar

to making votives.

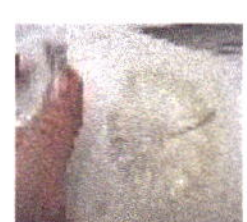

**Step 1.** Melt down your choice of wax. Place your floater moulds on waxed paper lined surface to catch any spills. With your wax at the proper pouring temperature, fill your floater moulds to the lip of the mould.

**Step 2.** Once the wax begins to cool, as seen by a slight haze forming along the edges of the mould, place your pre-tabbed wick into the floater mould. The tab will "stick" to the congealed wax on the bottom when it touches. Care should be taken to position the tab roughly in the centre of the mould.

**Step 3.** When the wax has completely cooled, it will have shrunken a bit, leaving a sink hole. To fix this, melt down saved wax from first pour, and heat it up 10 – 15 degrees hotter than the initial pour. This will allow proper adhesion between layers. Once your wax is at proper temperature, fill the mould again to the lip of the mould. You can also use a heat gun to smooth and even out the top of the floater.

**Step 4.** When the floaters are completely cool, and the tops are flattened out, remove them from the mould. They will usually slide right out without difficulty if they are completely cool. If you attempt to take them out too soon they will be more difficult to finally get them out.

## Making Container Candles

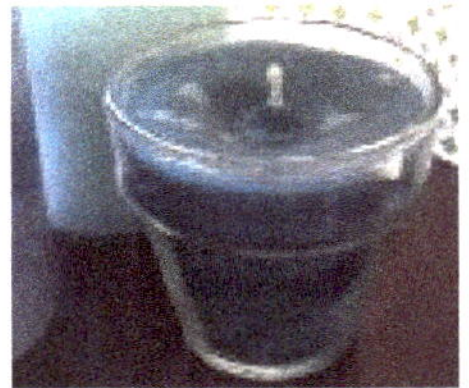

Essentially a container candle is a non-flammable container with wax and a wick. They have several advantages that make them popular. First of all, they are a bit like a candle and a candle holder rolled into one. They never drip, and because they are in a container; we can get away with using a lower melting point wax that enhances scent throw. That fact alone gives scented container candles the ability to effectively throw more scent than their free standing counterparts.

There are probably as many different ways to make container candles as there are candle makers. Soy, Palm, Paraffin or a blend of waxes are suitable for container candles and you may need to adjust some of the instructions below to achieve the results you want.

**Step 1. Prepare your Molten Wax Mixture**. You should be able to review these instructions while your wax is melting. Before continuing, set up a double boiler to melt your wax. A good target temperature is 170 – 175 degree F (77 °C - 80 °C) for a general wax. Once your wax has completely melted, add any additives you have selected and mix thoroughly. Add them in the following order:

1. Additives such as vybar or stearic acid (stearin), not needed in all the types of waxes
2. Dye
3. Fragrance oil (this is put in last so as to reduce the loss of the oil from the wax).

While your wax is melting, proceed through the next few steps. But, frequently keep an eye on your wax temperature.

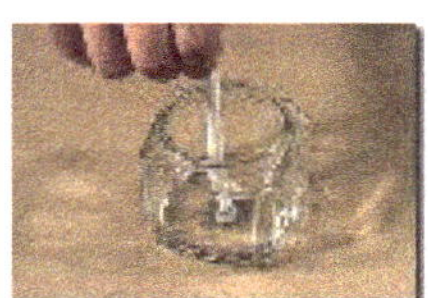

**Step 2. Add pre- tabbed Wicks to your Containers**. Disassemble a "Bic" pen or similar. Keep the barrel and discard the rest. Straighten your pre- tabbed wicks out. They don't have to be perfectly straight.

Insert the pre-tabbed wick through the barrel of the pen. 150mm wicks are good for this. If you have a different length, you may have to improvise. The point is the barrel makes handling the wick much easier.

While holding the wick within the barrel, apply hot-glue to the base of the wick tab. You can use a glue pot or a hot-glue gun for this. Another way is to use a small amount of blue tack on the bottom of the tab.

Using the barrel to guide the wick, press the tab to the centre of your container.

Slide the barrel off the wick. Proceed to the next step.

**Step 3. Secure the Top of your Wick**. Using a clothes pin, secure the top of your wick, so that the wick is central on the top of the container. Clothes pins are great for up to 75mm containers, bigger than that you will have to improvise. Looping the wick around a wooden skewer also works.

The objective here is to provide some sort of support to help keep the wick centered while the wax is cooling. You can actually carry out this step after you have poured the wax.

**Step 4.** Pre-heat your Container. Once your wax mixture is at the proper temperature, and you have thoroughly mixed in any additives, pre-heat your container to about 150 deg F (66 °C). You can use a heat gun or put the container in an oven set at the lowest setting. Exercise some care as heat guns can get much hotter than 150 deg F (66 °C).

**Note:** This step is not absolutely necessary, but it does improve the finished product. It permits us to pour our wax at a lower temperature without trapping bubbles and it improves the glass adhesion.

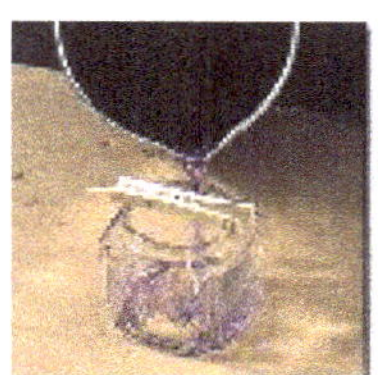

**Step 5. Initial Pour**. With your wax at the proper temperature 160 deg F (71°C), carefully fill your container the desired level. If it is a container with a lid, remember to fill it only to a level that will leave enough room for the lid to properly fit back on the finished candle.

Save about 20 percent of the wax in the pouring jug for step 6. Do NOT return it to the heat source.

Allow the wax to completely cool before proceeding. This will typically be six or more hours. Slow cooling generally provides the best results when it comes to container candles. So, don't attempt to accelerate the cooling process.

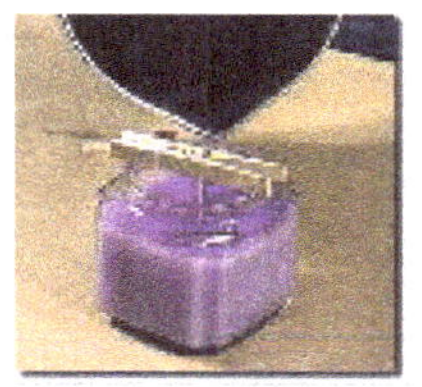

**Step 6. Re-pour**. Once your candle has completely cooled, you will notice that the wax has sunken a bit in the middle.

With the wax that you saved from the previous step, melt it back down and bring it to temperature of 185 deg F (85 °C). We use a higher temperature for the second pour because it increases the adhesion between the layers of wax.

Re-pour to a level that just barely covers the wax from the initial pour. Going to this level helps hide any seam lines.

Allow your candle to completely cool.

**Step 7. Trim Wick**. Once your candle has completely cooled, remove the clothe peg and trim the wick to 6mm.

### Making Chunk Candles

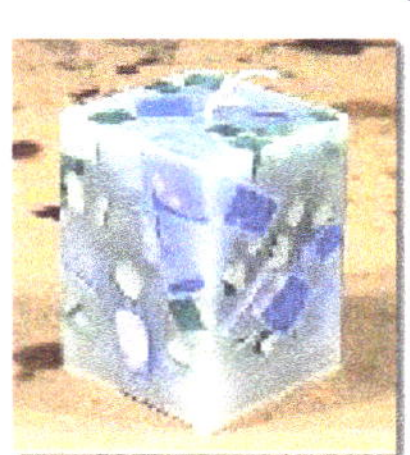

In addition to the normal items required for standard pillar candles, you will need the following items:

1. Baking tray with about a 12mm lip
2. Silicone spray

3. Utility knife or small pouring knife

4. Suggested wax Palm wax

**Step 1. Melt wax and add dye and fragrance oil as desired.**

Colour suggestions: Work with colours that are complimentary, generally those that occur together in nature. To find out what those are, look at any nature calendar. Also, keep in mind that you can dye the over-pour wax if desired. There are an infinite number of options at your disposal.

Using a double boiler and a thermometer, melt your wax and bring it to a temperature of about 190 deg F (88 °C). Add any additives, dye and fragrance oil that you have chosen and mix in well. You can scent and dye the chunks, the over-pour wax or both.

For this project, I have selected palm wax to make the chunks as well as the over-pour.

**Step 2. Grease a baking Tray.** To prevent the chunks from sticking to the baking tray, apply a thin film of non-sticking cooking spray of silicone spray. Either one will work. Wipe out the excess with a paper towel and leave only a very thin film.

A seasoned baking tray will not require anything to aid the release. Also, if you added fragrance oil to the wax, it will act as a release agent. Therefore you will not need any spray.

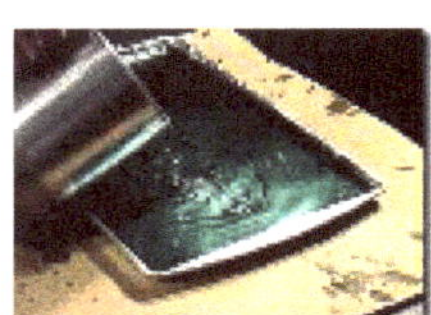

**Step 3. Pour wax into the Baking Tray.** With your wax at about 190 deg F (88 °C), pour it into the tray. Try not to spill or splatter. Pour the wax back and forth to distribute the heat throughout the tray. Pour to a depth that you would like your chunks to be. If you want small chunks, pour shallow. For large chunks, pour deeper.

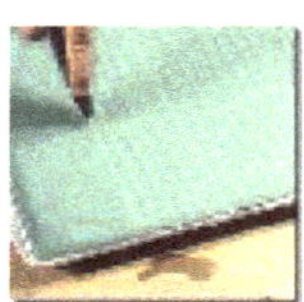

**Step 4. Slice the Chunks.** Allow the wax to cool to a point that it is firm but still pliable. It will be about the consistency of biscuit dough. Then, using a paring knife or utility knife, slice the wax into chunks. A criss-cross pattern works well.

This is an excellent opportunity for many other cookie cutter embeds - like stars, gingerbread men etc.

**Step 5. Remove the Chunks from the Baking Tray.** Allow the wax to completely cool. For this step, the more brittle it is the better. You may even want to chill the baking tray in the refrigerator, or outside if it is cool enough. Then flip it over and whack in onto a sheet of newspaper or waxed paper.

Most of the chunks should come apart. If some are still sticking together, they can be snapped apart by hand.

At this point you may want to make more chunks, even different colors.

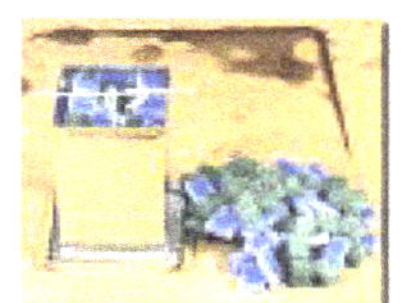

**Step 6. Fill the Mould with Chunks.** Wick your mold as usual (refer to pillar instructions). Then fill the prepared mould with chunks. You can arrange them nice and neat, or just drop them in any old how.

You can get creative by layering different colours. Also, you can use the chunks to pin embeds against the side walls of the mould. (Looks great).

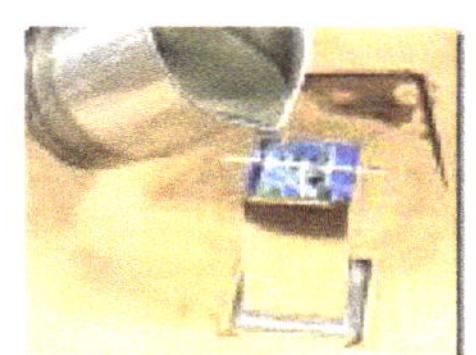

**Step 7. Fill with Over-pour Wax.** Heat your over-pour wax up to about 190 deg F (88 °C). Pour the wax into the mould to just cover the chunks.

Again you can add dye, fragrances, and additives to the over-pour wax if desired. Use a fairly translucent wax as the over-pour to allow the chunks to show through the wax a bit.

Optionally, you may vary the temperature of the over-pour. By increasing the temperature, you get the chunks to bleed a little. By lowering the temperature, you can introduce bubbles and surface texture.

Another option is to fill the mould only to the base of the chunks on the surface. The finished candle would then have chunks protruding through the top of the top. (Candle would be in a top- up orientation versus the typical top-down finish).

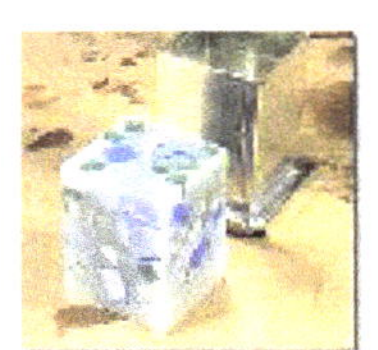

**Step 8. Remove the Chunk Candle from the mould.** Allow the candle to completely cool in the mould. This may take several hours depending on the size of the mould.

Chunk candles typically do not form too much of a sink hold. Therefore, re-pours are not necessary. Once it has cooled remove the finished candle form the mould.

### Making Balloon Luminaries

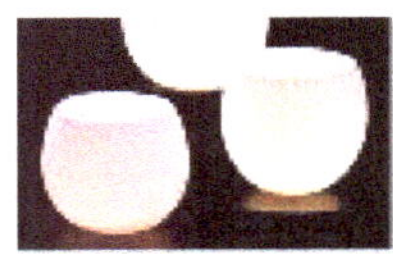

For a fun and easy project with a beautiful payoff, make these Balloon Luminaries.

You will need:

1. High melt wax
2. Water balloons
3. Double boiler
4. Wax sheet

**Step 1.** Fill a water balloon with tepid water

**Step 2.** Melt the wax. Optimum working temperature for this project is 180 deg F (82 °C). Try to maintain this temperature for your wax while working by keeping in on the double boiler.

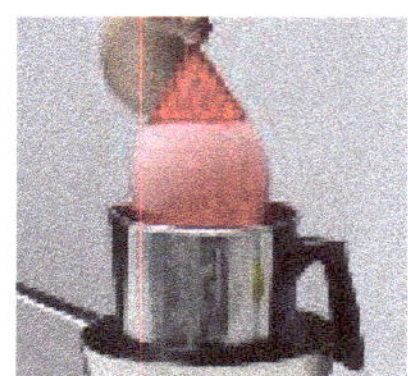

**Step 3.** Slowly dip your balloon into the wax to just below the water level in the balloon. **Warning: DO NOT dip the balloon into the wax past the water level. This may cause the balloon to burst.**

**Step 4.** Hold the balloon in the wax for a few seconds, and then slowly lift it out of the wax. Dip the balloon a few more times, allowing sometime between dips to let the wax to cool.

**Step 5.** While it is still quite warm carefully set the balloon down onto the piece of waxed paper, making sure that it is level. This will create a flat bottom for the luminary.

**Step 6.** Dip the balloon a few more times until it is the desired thickness. A good target thickness is 6 12mm. (¼ - ½”).

**Step 7.** Set the balloon on the paper again and let cool.

**Step 8**. When the wax is completely cooled, hold the balloon over a sink or bucket, facing away from you. Carefully pop the balloon with a skewer or knife and let the water drain out. Discard the burst balloon.

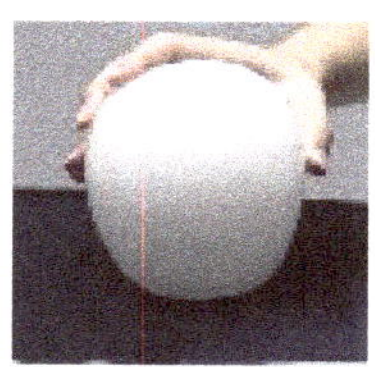

**Step 9**. To level the balloon luminary, heat a baking tray on the stove and place luminary top down onto the hot tray and carefully melt the edges until level.

**Step 10.** Place a Tea Light or Votive inside the luminary and burn on a candle holder in a dark area.

### Making Hurricane Shells

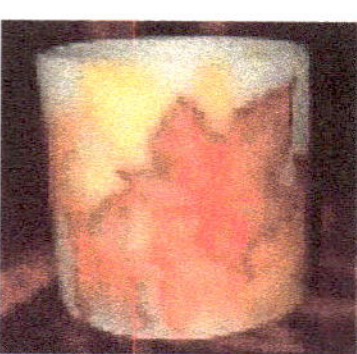

In addition to the normal items required for standard pillar candles, you will need the following items:

1. High melt wax with a melting point above 150 deg F (65.56 °)
2. A mould with a diameter of 100mm (4”) or wider
3. Hurricane insert or sleeve
4. Silicone spray or similar
5. Embedment’s, if desired
6. A utility knife or small paring knife

Many items may be used as embedments for hurricanes, such as:

- Dried botanicals

- Glass beads
- Wax chunks
- Silk flowers

**Step 1. Melt Wax and add Dye and / or Additives.** Using a double boiler and a thermometer, melt the wax and bring it to a temperature of about 190 deg F (87.78 °C). You will need to melt enough wax to fill your mould.

**Step 2. Set up a Water Bath.** Set up water bath, using either a sink or bucket. This step is not entirely necessary, but will speed things up dramatically and will produce a better finished product.

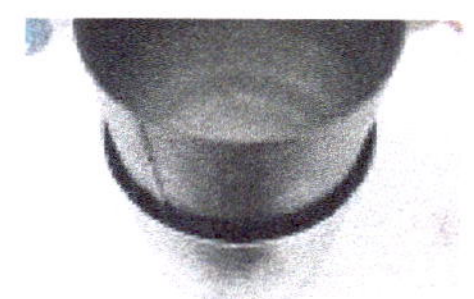

**Step 3. Prepare your Mould.** If the mould you select has a wick hole cover it with metal tape or mouldsealer.

You may wish to lightly coat the interior of your mould with silicone or cooking spray to aid in removing the finished shell. After spraying, wipe out any excess with a paper towel, leaving only a light film to coat the interior of the mould.

If you are using a hurricane insert, place it insider the mould. Then surround the insert with the embedments of your choice, taking care to arrange them how you would like them to appear in the finished candle. The purpose of the insert is to hold embedments against the sidewalls of the mould just long enough for them to adhere to the wax that will eventually solidify around them.

If you are not embedding anything in the walls of the shell, then you do not need the insert.

If you are using a water bath (and you should be), attach the appropriate weights to the bottom of the mould to stop it from floating.

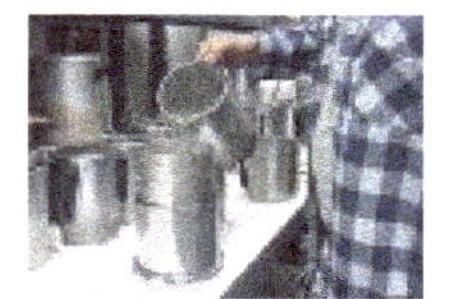

**Step 4. Pour Wax.** Double check your wax temperature to make sure that it is around 190 deg F (87.78 °C).

Pour the wax down into the centre of the mould insert. You may have to lift the insert slightly off the bottom of the mould to allow the hot wax to run up the side. Fill the mould to the height that you would like the finished candle to be. Generally, it is best to cover your embedments by at least 6mm.

Once filled, wait a minute or two and tap the sides of the metal mould with a blunt object, such as a wooden spoon, to free up any air bubbles and not damage the mould at the same time.

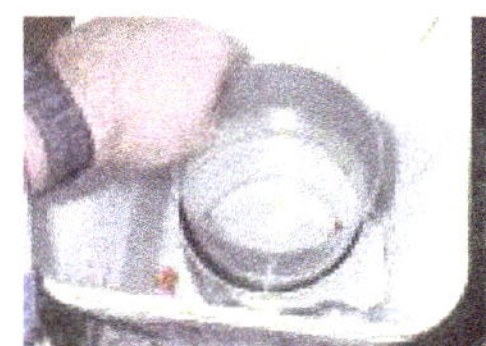

**Step 5. Place in Water Bath.** Carefully lower the mould into the water bath. The mould is very hot at this point, as is the wax inside it. Gloves or oven mitts come in handy here.

During cooling, lift the insert slightly off the bottom about every 2 – 3 minutes. This will prevent the insert from becoming embedded in the cooling wax on the bottom of the mould.

The wax will cool from the exterior and begin to solidify inwards. Once you are confident that all embedments are being held in place by the solidifying wax, remove the insert completely.

With the insert removed, allow the side walls to continue to solidify. Once the sidewalls are about 12mm thick, remove the mould from the water bath. It takes only about 20 minutes in a water bath to form a shell of the proper thickness.

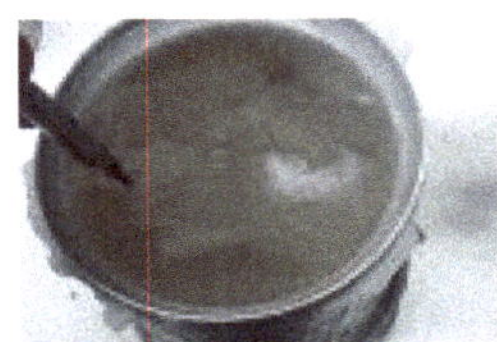

**Step 6. Pour out Inner Wax**. Remove any weights from the mould. Quickly dry the exterior with a paper towel to remove any excess water.

The surface of the wax may have formed a skin. Using a knife slice an opening all the way around the top. You will want to slice at a position that is just at the inner edge of the sidewalls. Scoop out the skin with a spoon before it sink to the bottom, or else it will quickly stick to the bottom.

In one quick, smooth action, dump the inner liquid wax back into the melting pot.

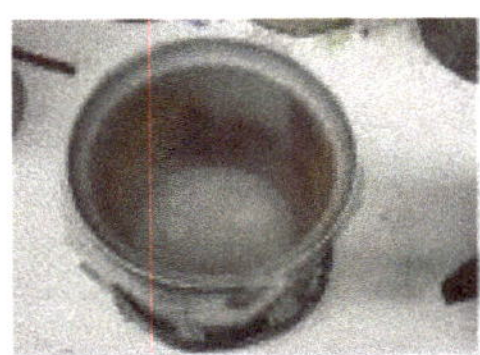

**Step 7. Remove from Mould.** Allow the hurricane shell to completely cool before attempting to remove it from the mould. Trying to remove it too early is likely to result in a cracked shell, or a marred exterior. Be patient.

If the hurricane shell doesn't slide out of the mould easily, then try chilling it in the refrigerator for about 20 minutes.

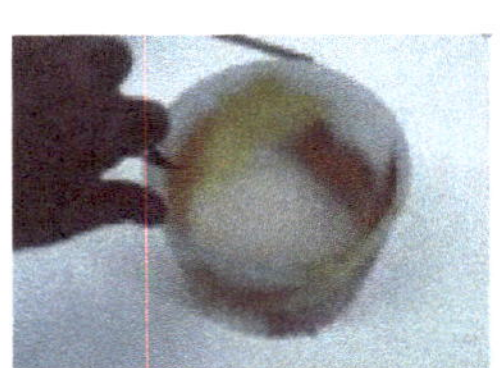

**Step 8. Level the Top.** Place a baking tray on top of simmering water. The hated tray can then be used to melt away some of the wax on the top of the hurricane shell. Level the top to provide a clean appearance. If you have an electric griddle/frypan, you may wish to use it on low heat.

You also may use a paring knife to help trim away any sharp edges.

**Step 9. Insert Votive.** Place a votive holder containing a votive candle inside your finished hurricane shell. Or, you may use a small container candle (votivesize).

### Embedding Photos in Candles

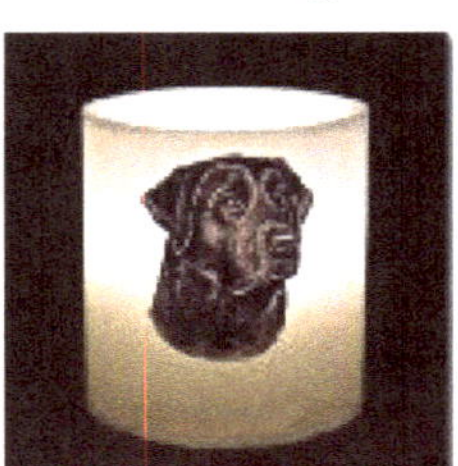

Any image that you can print on paper will work. This opens a plethora of opportunities for embedding various artistic designs and illustrations.

In addition to the normal items required for standard pillar candles, you will need the following items:

1. High melt straight wax with a melting point above 150 deg F (65.56 °)

2. A mould with a diameter of 100mm (4") or wider (wider the better)
3. Mould weights
4. Water bath
5. Wet wash cloth
6. An image printed on plain paper

Embedding photos in candles is not as hard as it might seem. If you'd like to share keepsake photos in a unique and charming way, this is a great way to do it. The largest obstacle in embedding photos in candles is probably getting the photos close enough to the surface so that you may clearly see what is depicted. In pursuit of getting photos to appear as clearly as possible, many people have resolved to use decoupage or water-slide decals to affix images on to the exterior of the candle. In contrast, these instructions will demonstrate a very simple technique to secure an embedded photo directly against the exterior surface of the candle so that it is clearly visible, but is still fully integrated into the wax. For those that might be interested in offering this service as part of their candle making business, the results are reproducible and predictable enough that you could put these out in volumes if desired.

We'll start by looking at what to actually embed. Don't embed the actual photo. Instead, scan the photo and put it in digital format and print it out. My suggestion is to use just plain copy/printer paper. Heavier paper will obstruct the passage of light. Once you have got it printed, crop it so that it will fit into the mould you're planning to use. Also, consider the possibility of doing a cutout in a fashion where you'll end up with a silhouette. Sometimes it's nice that way, other times it is not.

In these instructions we will be embedding the photo in a hurricane shell. However, the same principles could be applied to embedding photos in a regular pillar candle. When embedding photos in pillar candles, care must be taken in selecting a wick size that will not produce enough heat to create a fire hazard with the embedded photos. My suggestion is to use a wick of the smallest size possible. Also, use a high melting point wax to further suppress the flame. Then burn it only for a short time before filling the created cavity with a tea light for lasting enjoyment. As always test your finished product for safety.

**Step 1. Prepare water bath.** Begin by preparing your mould for the water bath. A water bath will be needed in this project. In preparation for the water bath, attach weights to the mould. Also, prepare a water vessel with the appropriate amount of water.

**Step 2. Melt Wax**. Because this is a hurricane shell and we want it to withstand the heat without melting, we are using a high melting point wax. The melting point of the wax used in this project is about 163 deg F (72.78 °C). My suggestion is to use a wax with a melting point above 150 deg F (65.56 °C); the higher, the better.

3 tablespoons of stearic acid (stearin) per 0.45kg (1lb) of wax was used to increase the opacity (whiteness) of the wax. Stearic acid is entirely optional when using high melting point waxes that already possess some opacity. No fragrances or dyes are used.

Melt your wax to 185-190 deg F (85 °- 87.78 °C). Please review wax melting instructions and pay attention to the safety advice.

**Step 3. Pour the wax into Mould.** If the mould you select has a wick hole, plug it some metal tape or mould sealer.

You may wish to lightly coat the interior of your mould with silicone or cooking spray to aid in removing the finished shell. After spraying, wipe out any excess with a paper towel, leaving only a light film to coat the interior of the mould.

With the wax temperature is at around 190 deg F (87.78 °C). Fill the mould.

I always fill my molds to a point no higher than about 12mm from the top of the mould. The 12mm clearance minimises the possibility of spillage, when you later have to move the mould, e.g. to or from the waterbath.

**Step 4. Submerge Photo into Wax.** Insert your photo into the wax filled mould. Fully submerge the photo and allow it to sit for a moment or two. It will soak up wax and displace any air that is within the paper.

If there are bubbles still sticking to the photo, try to move the photo around a bit to dislodge as many of the bubbles as possible. Chopsticks are very handy for this operation. Having no bubbles is ideal. However, not always practicable, don't waste too much time on this step.

Also, lightly tap the side of the mould with a blunt object to free up any bubbles that may still be there.

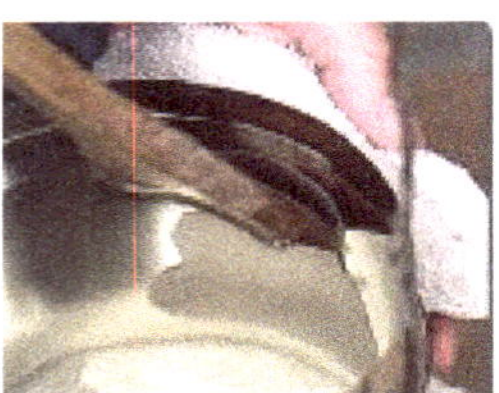

**Step 5. Position the Photo using a spoon and a wet cloth.** Whilst using the utensils of your choice, position the photo against the sidewall of the mould. A wooden spoon that is preheated in the hot wax is good for this. If the spoon was cold, the photo would stick to it on contact.

With the photo in place, take a wet towel or such like and apply it to the exterior of the mould at the location of the photo.

The wet cloth will absorb heat from the wax and it should solidify around the photo fairly quickly. You may have to rotate the cloth to use cooler parts of it as needed. The frost that forms inside around the photo is solidified wax that will secure the photo in place long enough to get the mould into the water bath.

**Step 6. Place the mould in the water bath.** The entire interior will frost up right away.

When the shell is as thick as you'd like it to be, remove the mould from the water bath. 9-12mm (3/8 - 1/2") is a goodtarget thickness.

Step 7. Pour out inner Wax. Remove any weights from the mould. Quickly dry the exterior with a paper towel to remove any excess water.

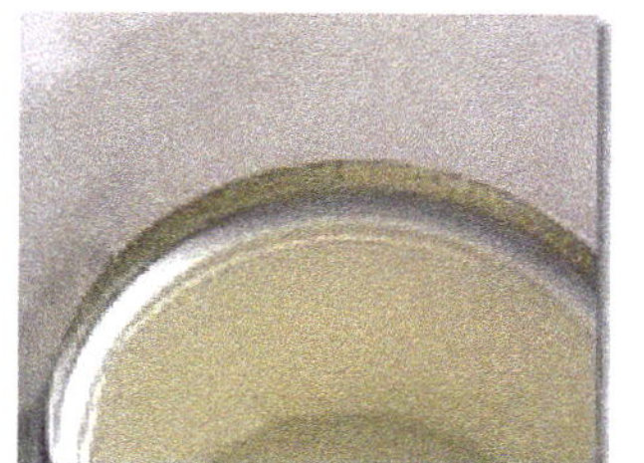

The surface of the wax may have formed a skin. Using a knife slice an opening all the way around the top. You will want to slice at a position that is just at the inner edge of the sidewalls. Scoop out the skin with a spoon before it sink to the bottom, or else it will quickly stick to the bottom.

In one quick, smooth action, dump the inner liquid wax back into the melting pot.

Allow the hurricane shell to completely cool before attempting to remove it from the mould. Trying to remove it too early is likely to result in a cracked shell, or a marred exterior. Be patient.

If the hurricane shell doesn't slide out of the mould easily, then try chilling it in the refrigerator for about 20 minutes.

**Step 8. Level the Top.** Place a baking tray on top of simmering water. The heated tray can then be used to melt away some of the wax on the top of the hurricane shell. Level the top to provide a clean appearance. If you have an electric griddle/frypan, you may wish to use it on low heat.

You also may use a paring knife to help trim away any sharp edges.

**Step 9. Insert Votive.** Place a votive holder containing a votive candle inside your finished hurricane shell. Or, you may use a small container candle (votive size).

### Making Mosquito Repellant Candles

I seem to have the right blood for the mosquitoes as they love me. No matter who I'm with they come for me first. David Fisher, from About.com has some good recipes and ideas on how to make citronella candles. He also includes other suggested essential oils such as clove, cedar wood, lavender, eucalyptus and others.

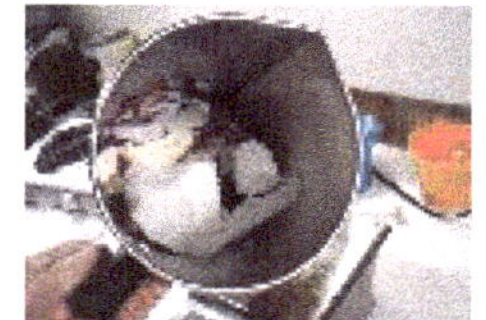

**Step 1. Get your equipment ready.** Like any candle project, get all of your supplies and materials ready before you start. A well-organized workshop is a safe workshop.

The great thing about outdoor citronella candles is that you don't want them to burn well. You want them to smoke a bit. It helps the mosquito repelling effect. Also, you want a big pool to help to disperse the essential oils. This is also a good project to use up all of the scrap wax.

**Step 2. Priming large Wicks.** For this project you will probably have to assemble and prime your own wicks. I suggest using MC-1 size wick for 100mm metal buckets.

To prime the wicks, cut them to the length and soak them in some melted wax for several minutes. You will see small bubbles streaming out of the wicks.

Stir the wax a bit and press on the wicks to make sure that the wax soaks in well. Lay the wicks out straight on a piece of paper to harden.

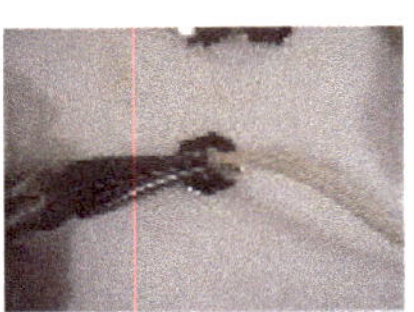

**Step 3. Assemble the Wicks.** Once the wicks are cooled, you can put the wick tab on the bottom of the wick. Using a pair of pliers, open up the hole in the wick tab, insert the wick through, and close the tabs onto thewick.

Using a glue dot or a dab of hot glue, position the wick tab in the centre of the bottom of the bucket.

**Step 4. Melt the Wax and add the Essential oils.** Melt the wax in a double boiler. Most container waxes want to be heated to about 175 deg F (79.44 °C).

Add your essential oil blend and stir well.

You can usually use about 1oz (28.35gr) for every 1lb (0.45kg). You can vary this up or down depending on the blend and how strong you want it. You probably don't want to go much above 1.5oz (42.52gr) per 1lb (0.45kg) of wax. More than this and you could affect the burning of the candle and also, the cost of the candle will rapidly increase.

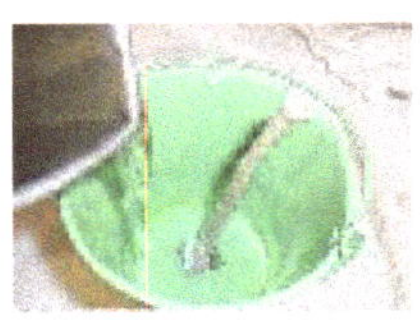

**Step 5. Pour the Wax.** Let the wax cool to about 160 deg F (71 °C), gently stirring as it cools. Pour the wax into the bucket.

Use sticks or skewers to help keep the wick centered. Put the candles in a safe place to cool.

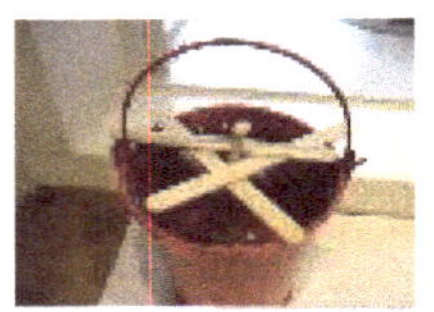

Once the candles have cooled for at least 24 hours, it's time to light them up. Don't forget to take notes on how the wicks, wax and essential oils perform.

***Note:*** *Be sure to use extra caution with these candles. The large wicks produce large flames and melt pools. Be sure to place them where people, children and animals will not bump into them or knock them over. And never use them indoors.*

Don't settle for just plain old citronella oil. There are a number of widely available essential oils that are reputed to help repel mozzies including: Clove, cedar wood, lavender, eucalyptus, peppermint, rosemary, lemongrass and others.

These oils you can blend in with citronella in just about any combination you want.

# Questions & Answers

**Q.** I've just started a new hobby Candle making and I want to know what else can I use to melt the beeswax, because I don't have a double boiler?

**A.** Believe it or not, you may already have a double boiler in your home right now. If you have two pots - no matter how large or small - which fit one inside the other and you are able to put some water in the larger pot, then the beeswax in the smaller one.

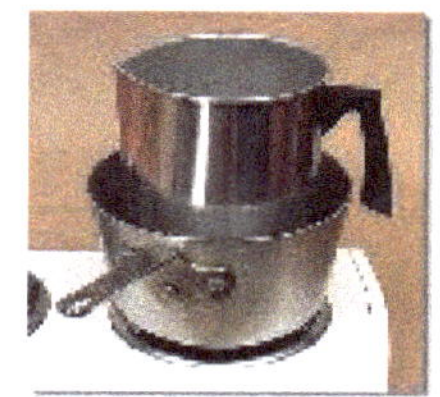

Then put the smaller pot with the beeswax inside the larger pot with the water, turn on the heat and you have a double boiler. You DO NOT want to put so much water in the larger one that you aren't able to have the smaller one be surrounded by the water. Notice I said "surrounded" and not submerged. The weight of the pot and the beeswax will automatically seek its own level.

**Q.** How do I calculate the burn time of my candles?

**A.** Before you light the candle use a scale to weigh it. Once you have the original weight trim the wick and light the candle, letting it burn for four hours. When the four hours are up blow it out, let it cool, and weigh it again. Subtract the weight after the burn cycle from the original weight and divide by the number of hours. The number you end up with is your hourly burn rate.

Once you have the hourly burn weight divide the weight of the whole candle* by the hourly rate and you end up with the number of hours your candle will burn.

**Amount Consumed** (Original wt. - wt. After Burning) ÷ **Hours Burnt** = **Hourly Burn Rate Original wt.** (minus wt. of container) ÷ **Hourly Burn Rate** = **Approximate Burn Time**

If you are testing a container candle make sure to subtract the weight of the container from the weight of the whole candle before dividing by your hourly rate.

Ounces work fine for calculating the burn rate but if your scales have grams as an option, we would recommend using that. Since grams are so much smaller than ounces you end up with nicer numbers (5 grams/hr. instead of .16 ounces/hr.).

Although one burn cycle (four hours) will give you a fairly accurate hourly burn rate numerous cycles (three or four) will produce a much more accurate number. The first burn cycle is always a little off because the wick is not yet completely saturated with wax, color, and fragrance.

Q. How much wax will my mold hold?

A. Although different waxes have varying densities we have put together a quick formula based on diameter and height to calculate how much wax you will need.

Here are the weights per inch of a round candle:

- 2 inch diameter = 38 grams or 1.35 ounces per inch
- 3 inch diameter = 100 grams or 3.5 ounces per inch
- 4 inch diameter = 165 grams or 5.8 ounces per inch

So, say you have a 6 1/2 inch round pillar mold and you need to know how much wax you will need to make a candle.

You would use the 3 inch diameter rate per inch (3.5 ounces) times the height (6.5 inches).

3.5 X 6.5 = 22.75 ounces of wax to make the candle.

Q. Can fragrance oils be used in oil warmers?

**A.** Yes.

**Q.** What does the fragrance flashpoint mean?

**A.** The flashpoint is the temperature at which fragrances can combust if exposed to open flame or spark. Adding fragrance oil to wax that is above the flashpoint will not cause it to combust. With fragrance at room temperature and no flame there is no cause for concern.

Do low flashpoint fragrances burn off? No. As long as fragrance is added to wax and poured soon it will not lose strength. However, we do not recommend repeatedly cooling and reheating batches of fragranced wax. Limiting your batch size to an amount you can pour right away is always better.

So why list flashpoint at all? Flashpoints are listed for two reasons; customers who make gel candles, and air shipments. The recommended use is for fragrances with flashpoints over 170° F in gel waxes. Plus we are unable to ship fragrances with low flashpoints via air.

**Q.** What are the advantages of Palm Wax?

**A.** Palm wax has a very beautiful and unique look, throws fragrance incredibly well, and is a one- pour for containers, votives and pillars.

**Appearance**: Palm wax is truly striking. It has a unique pattern and pearlescence that people remember.

**Fragrance Throw**: A palm candle can fill a room, or even a house, with less fragrance than you may think. Using candle science fragrance oils, we've found that 3-6% (1/2 to 1oz/lb.) yields fragrance throw that is truly impressive. Find out more on our Fragrance & Palm page.

**Single Pour**: With a little care, palm is a true one pour in containers AND in votives and pillars. This totally unique attribute means less time and better looking candles.

**Q.** Email being sent around the web. Subject: Gel Candles

*You don't use Gel Candles, do you? I received this from a friend of mine and wanted to make you aware of this terrible episode with candles.*

*Thought this might be of some news to you!*

*Hi all, my former secretary had a terrible thing happen to her and her family last week, and I wanted to share it with all of you so that you could be warned and warn your friends and family as well.*

*She had a gel candle burning in her bathroom...it exploded and caught her house on fire...the house burned down and they have lost everything. The fire marshal told her that this is not the first incident where a gel candle has exploded and caused a fire. He said that the gel builds up a gas, and often times it explodes and sets fire to the room it is in, which is what happened to her. The fire was so hot it melted the smoke alarm, and they did not discover the fire until there was an explosion, which was her toilet blowing up, and then it was too late...the entire upstairs was engulfed in flames.*

*Smoke damage and water damage have destroyed what wasn't destroyed by fire. I know that there are roomies and friends that I don't have on this list because I can't remember how to spell their screen names...please pass this along to anyone I missed. I would not want this to happen to anyone else.*

*Her family is devastated. All their mementos and everything of value and meaning are gone. I'm not trying to bring anyone down...just a friendly warning to all of you about the use of gel candles left unattended.*

*Thanks and take care!*

*NOTE: Marty and I know a lady who loves the gel candles. She had one burning on her mantle and it caught fire just like in the message above.*

*She was at home at the time and saw it happen and grabbed the candle to keep it from setting her home on fire and it came apart in her hand. She saved her home but suffered 3rd degree burns to her hand and 3 fingers!*

*Please, if you or anyone you know have these candles, don't light them, they*

*are dangerous. Please, pass this on. God Bless.*

**A.** That e-mail that you sent is a chain letter type of mail that's been circulating around the web for months now. I don't know where it started or who wrote it, and there is no way to know or prove if there's any truth to it. In fact that letter is even listed on the Urban Legends & Web lore site, check out this link:

http://urbanlegends.about.com/science/urbanlegends/library/blgelcandles.htm?iam=dpile&terms=%2Bgel+%2Bcandle+%2Bdanger

I do believe that it is definitely an exaggeration if not total fiction. Gel does not produce any "gas" that I'm aware of, and I don't see any way it could possibly "blow up" a toilet. The problem here is misinformation. It's not that gel candles produce some kind of gas in the air; the problem is that some gel candles are not made properly and with the correct type of supplies, so they can be unsafe. The most common cause of a gel fire is use of the wrong type of fragrance oil in the gel. Polar fragrance oils can separate from the gel and form pockets, which can cause the candle to burn improperly or possibly flare up in spots. If the oil is a low flash point, it is more likely to flare up, and it also lowers the overall flash point of the finished product to an unsafe level.

Also, gel does burn hotter than regular wax, so great care must be taken to use only thick, quality heat resistant glassware that won't shatter when burning. Candles don't "explode" so to speak, but they can crack or shatter if they get too hot and the glassware is too thin. The third problem is, even as it mentions in that story, that people are leaving their candles burning unattended in another room. Consumers need to start reading the caution labels and taking it seriously.

Gel candlemakers need to study and research and be sure to use only the correct types of supplies so they produce safe gel candles, and they need to test burn their products before putting them on the market. It's unfortunate that there are so many unsafe candles on the market that it's giving all candles a bad reputation.

**Q.** I am not getting a good scent throw in my candles. Could it be the fragrance?

**A.** We understand that scent throw issues can be frustrating to you. However, approximately 98% of the time when using a reputable company for your supplies, scent throw problems in candles are not caused by the fragrance. There are several things that can inhibit scent throw: Using soy wax, not using a hot enough burning wick, using too much color, using too much vybar, adding fragrance to wax at too hot of a temperature, and not allowing candles to cure (set for several days after you make them).

**Q.** I notice that with some of my fragrances, I cannot get the candle to get a full melt-pool across the top. Why?

**A.** Fragrances vary in flash point and specific gravity. When a fragrance has a high flash point and high specific gravity, it requires a hotter burning wick to allow the fragrance to evaporate out of the wax, and to get a nice melt-pool. When a fragrance has a low flash point and low specific gravity, it requires a smaller sized wick to allow the fragrance to evaporate out of the wax, and get a nice melt- pool. Vanilla fragrances tend to require a hotter burning wick; while citrus fragrances will require a smaller sized wick.

**Q**. How do I get my wicks to stay in place while my container candles are cooling?

**A.** To prevent your wicks from falling over while the candle is cooling, we suggest you use hair combs. Simply secure your wick in the bristles of the comb, and lay the comb on top of the container.

**Q.** After burning my candles, I notice black clumps on top of my wick. How can I avoid this?

**A.** All wicks produce carbon "mushrooming" when burning. Some wicks produce less mushrooming than others. Since carbon is let off whenever something is burned, we do not know how to prevent mushrooming from occurring.

**Q.** Can I use your soy wax in cosmetic products?

**A.** Yes, as long as the soy wax is 100% soy wax. It is also considered Kosher, and is safe enough to eat. Soy wax can be added to your cosmetic products.

**Q**. How can I increase my scent throw in my soy wax candles?

**A.** The molecular structure of soy wax contains various types of chemical bonds that make it harder to break down than paraffin wax. Its structure is more prone to trapping scent, than allowing it to evaporate freely. It takes more heat to break down these chemical bonds; therefore, you will need to use hotter burning wicks when making soy candles. Try increasing your wick size. Also, we suggest that you use 1.5 ounces of fragrance per pound of soy wax with the majority of our fragrances. If you are still not happy with the scent throw of your soy wax candles, consider using a soy/paraffin blend wax. Joy wax may be the answer to your problems."

**Q.** My soy wax candle tops are frosted looking. How can I prevent this from occurring?

**A.** Soy wax will naturally have a frosted look on the tops of candles; however, you can reduce the amount of frosting by pouring your candle wax at 100-115 degrees. At this temperature, your wax will be slushy in appearance.

**Q.** What causes a candle to smoke, and what can I do to correct it?

**A.** A well-made candle will create virtually no smoke when burning properly. However, if the wick becomes too long, or an air current disturbs the flames teardrop shape, small amounts of unburned carbon particles (soot) will escape from the flame as a visible wisp of smoke. Any candle will soot if the flame is disturbed.

To avoid this, always trim the wick to ¼ inch before every use and be sure to place candles away from drafts, vents or air currents. If a candle continually flickers or smokes, it is not burning properly and should be extinguished. Allow the candle to cool, trim the wick, make sure the area is draft free, and then re-light.

**Q.** Is my candle biodegradable?

**A.** Probably. Studies have shown that beeswax, paraffin and vegetable-based waxes are biodegradable. The vast majority of candles today are made primarily from these waxes.

Q. Are there any other types of candles to make?

A. Yes Go to www.soy4you.com and check the Hints &Tips section

## Troubleshooting

**Troubleshooting for Container and Moulded Candles**

| Problem | Solution |
|---|---|
| **There are lines inside the glass** | ▪ The glass wasn't heated prior to pouring wax |
| **The candle surface has bubbles** | ▪ The wax was too hot<br>▪ The wax was poured too quickly<br>▪ The wax was too cold when poured<br>▪ Use a heat gun or hair dryer to remove bubbles |
| **When burning the flame burns in a tunnel down the centre of candle** | ▪ The wick is too small, Ensure that you use the proper size wick based on the diameter of the container<br>▪ Candle didn't properly burn for one hour for every inch in diameter of container |
| **Chalky frosting on surface of candle** | ▪ Candle sat in a room temperature area and then placed in a much cooler area, Soy candles are |

| | |
|---|---|
| | very sensitive in extreme heat inside an oven or use heat gun |
| **The wick is smoking excessively** | ▪ The wick is too small and will not consume the melted wax<br>▪ Too much fragrance oil and some dyes can clog the wick |
| **Wick has moved after pouring wax** | ▪ Make sure you secure the wick to the base of the container using glue dots or similar. If the wax is too hot this will cause the glue dot to not adhere to the container |
| **The candle won't release from mould** | ▪ The mould could have dents<br>▪ The wax may not have completely cooled. Allow candle to completely cool for at least 24 hours<br>▪ The well was overfilled when topped-off to fill sink holes. Be sure not to go above the previous pour |

## Candle Forums

Listed below are technical forums you can visit or join to find questions to many of your candle problems, and to network with others doing what you do.

**Candle Tech**
www.candletech.com

**Moon Glow Soy Chat**
http://groups.yahoo.com/group/MoonGlowSoy/join

**The Candle Cauldron**
www.candle.cauldron.com

**Soy Wax Candles.Org**
www.forumcityusa.com/index.php?mforum=soywaxcandles

**The scent Review**
www.thescentreview.com/board

# Candle TestSheet

| | |
|---|---|
| Date | |
| Temp of Room | |
| Container Style | |
| Type of Wick(s) | |
| No. of Wicks | |
| Amount of fragrance (per lb/kg of wax) | |
| Wax Brand & Type | |
| Additives | |
| Pouring Temperature | |
| Jars Heated – Yes or No | |
| | |
| Cure Time | |
| Wet Spots | |
| Bubbles | |
| Frosting | |
| Cold Throw | |
| Hot Throw | |
| Burn & Scent Quality after 30 minutes | |
| Burn & Scent Quality after 1 Hour | |
| Burn & Scent Quality after 2 Hours | |
| Burn & Scent Quality after 3 Hours | |
| Burn & Scent Quality after 4 Hours | |
| Tunnelling Effect? | |
| Other | |

Additional Comments:

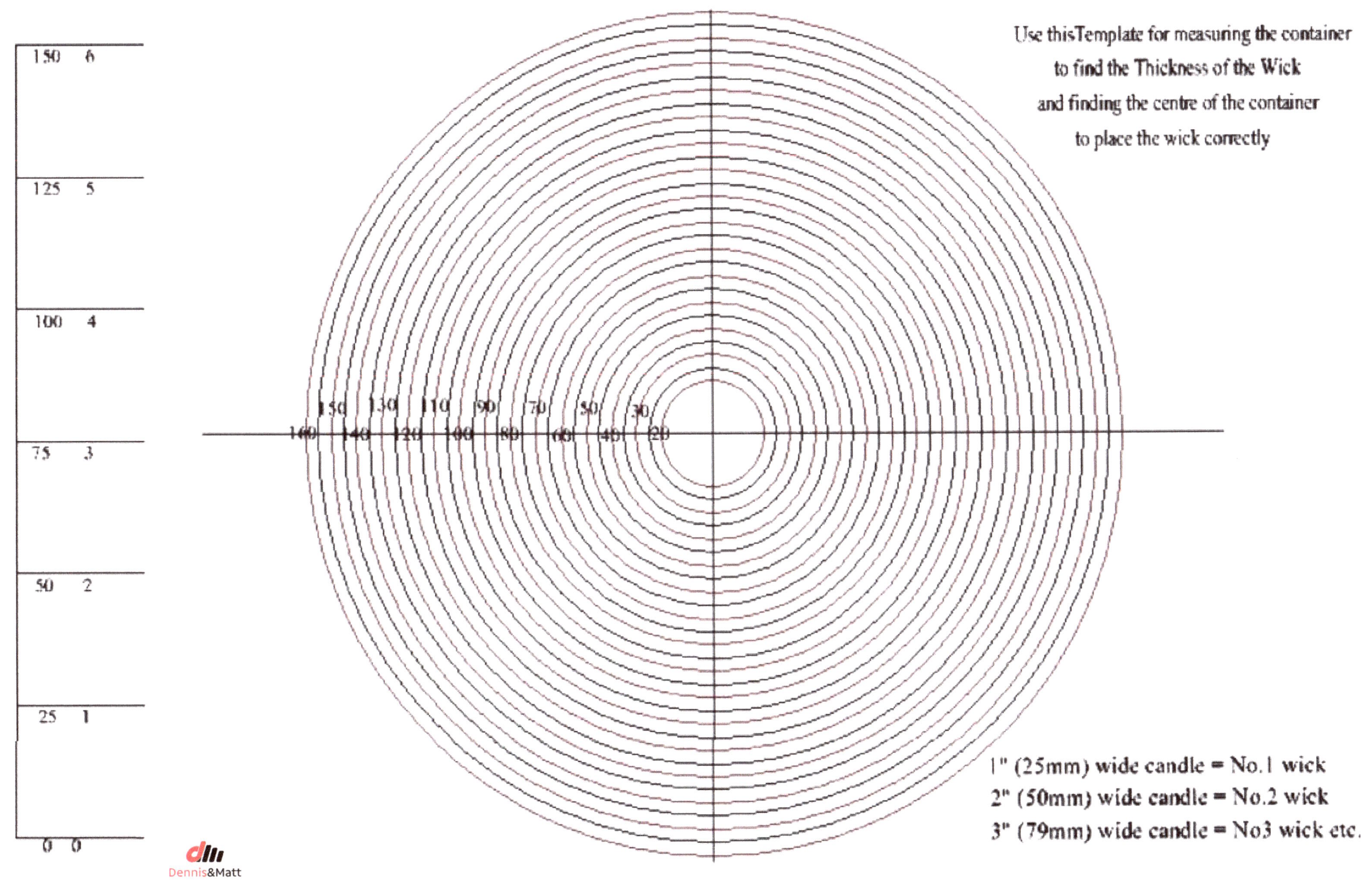

Use thisTemplate for measuring the container
to find the Thickness of the Wick
and finding the centre of the container
to place the wick correctly
150 6
125 5
100 4
75 3
50 2
25 1
0 0
160 150 140 130 120 110 100 90 80 70 60 50 40 30 20
1" (25mm) wide candle = No.1 wick
2" (50mm) wide candle = No.2 wick
3" (79mm) wide candle = No3 wick etc.
Dennis&Matt

www.ingramcontent.com/pod-product-compliance
Lightning Source LLC
Chambersburg PA
CBHW041414060826
49398CB00059B/689

*9781716619533*